Africa Focus Debates on Contemporary Contentious Biomedical Issues

Munyaradzi Mawere

Langaa Research & Publishing CIG
Mankon, Bamenda

Publisher
Langaa RPCIG
Langaa Research & Publishing Common Initiative Group
P.O. Box 902 Mankon
Bamenda
North West Region
Cameroon
Langaagrp@gmail.com
www.langaa-rpcig.net

Distributed in and outside N. America by African Books Collective
orders@africanbookscollective.com
www.africanbookcollective.com

ISBN: 9956-726-02-8

© Munyaradzi Mawere 2011

Dedication

To my aunt, Maria Machata, my brothers and sisters I humbly and gratefully dedicate this book, which you spiritually and morally initiated and nurtured until it has become a laudable reality.

Dedication

Table of Contents

vi

Preface

This book is a product of my imaginative forays into biomedicine related issues. It generally focuses on selected burning issues in contemporary medical ethics. In particular, the book critically examines four issues: euthanasia, physicians/medical doctors' strike, advertising in traditional medicine and the principle of beneficence in biomedicine. I will briefly explain how the book tackles each of these burning and/or contentious issues in contemporary medical ethics.

The first four chapters which make the bulk of this book examine the concept of euthanasia and the moral controversies surrounding it. The argument advanced in these chapters is that the intractable nature of euthanasia makes it at root ethical and, in part, cultural. It is in part cultural because it involves issues to do with beliefs, customs and traditions of individuals or a group of people. On the other hand, it is at root ethical because it concerns itself with human behaviour and conduct and the difference between right and wrong, good and bad. This denotes that euthanasia like the other three issues considered later in this book - physicians' strike, advertising in traditional medicine and the principle of beneficence- does not deal solely with factual judgments which can be said to be either true or false; hence its complexity. Consequently, the question on euthanasia has become a common game for almost everybody- moralists, economists, academicians, national governments and the public. It has also become one of the most contentious of the 21st century issues in the medical fraternity.

In the light of this observation, the first four chapters (of this book) conceptually analyses euthanasia, dismantles, rethink and reconstruct some of the arguments that have been forwarded by researchers over the years before it advances a "moderate view of euthanasia" and "the principle of negotiated justice". The chapters make an attempt to demonstrate through "hypothetical cases" and others drawn from real life situations the plausibility of a moderate view of euthanasia and the principle of negotiated justice associated with it. This view is useful in that it pays veneration to the sanctity of life while at the same time respects the patient's rights and promotes the majority's participation in the judgment of euthanasia cases. Thus the view employs an emancipator and democratic approach -negotiated justice-that represent a modern human right oriented response from a patient and the public's perspective. These approaches are pragmatic in so far as they use "exemplary cases" to demonstrate how we can seek to understand the impact of euthanasia from credence values of beneficence, mercy and simple logic. I believe the fruits of this intellectual inventory will be a blessing not just to the medical fraternity, but also to members of the public and medical ethics, which benefit immensely from the increasing availability of the treasure of literature on this controversial issue- euthanasia -rendered ethically and in ways conforming to the discursive parameters of scholarly works. In most if not all countries, the approach used in the first four chapters of this book comes as a necessity because in the name of euthanasia, unnecessary deaths and sufferings of the patients as well as the public are a common thing. And civil rights and individual rights are often violated and neglected at the expense of tradition and socio-political ideology, yet there are long term advantages to be gained by actively promoting them. The virtue of the first four chapters of this book thus, is to ascertain how useful and influential the "moderate view of euthanasia" is, especially as a strategy where forces of medical ethics would essentially benefit healthy professionals, patients, members of the public and their national governments in decision making relevant to the medical fraternity. In this view, it can be rightly asserted that the book is a contribution towards efforts by researchers in the field of medical ethics. It shifts emphasis from the dominant western view of euthanasia and the African traditional view of euthanasia to a more pragmatic and rationalized view.

Still on the first four chapters, perhaps it is worth mentioning that the book partly discusses euthanasia using a case study of sub-Saharan Africa heretofore referred to as Africa, not because euthanasia is an issue that affects the sub-Saharan Africa alone, but because it is one continent that has been drastically impacted by this issue, negatively or otherwise. Generally the African view of euthanasia needs serious examination, reconstitution and reconstruction or both. The main problem, however, is whether we can in any meaningful and coherent manner talk about an African view of euthanasia that covers or incorporates the inevitable nuances that go with cultural and individual differences of the African people in the continent and those in the Diaspora. I have adopted the principles of charity where in hermeneutical studies I am allowed to carry out my interpretation with some sense of liberalism and assumption which is not harmful to the spirit of interpretation and writing. As such, I have assumed that all Africans in the continent and those in the Diaspora are bound to have more in common than with people of other continents. Also, I have not pretended to say everything in African traditional culture(s) except that which directly intertwine with the theme of this book. I have used more examples common in some African countries than others, but making sure not to lose focus in my treatment of the view of euthanasia in sub-Saharan Africa as a whole.

Chapters 5, 6 and 7 respectively examine the controversies surrounding medical doctors/physicians' strikes, advertising in traditional medicine and the principle of beneficence in biomedicine. It is argued in this book that all these issues, as with euthanasia, are difficult to give a precise answer. The book however proffers various arguments and windows to/ways of examining these issues in order to arrive at the best possible answer to each case that arises in biomedicine. It is hoped that the arguments raised and ways (to deal with the problems) suggested in this book will be key to unlock and examine all controversial cases within the precincts of biomedicine.

For a majority of students of philosophy, medicine, anthropology and sociology, this book qualifies as food for thought and indeed a text they would enjoy reading. It shows them the wisdom that lies in "liberal thinking" and encourages them to start on the path of critical thinking and careful reasoning for themselves. The book, above all else, attempts to show that questioning and indeed right questioning matters most, not only in philosophy but other spheres of life. To this end, the book offers a subtle approach to debate and honest self-reflection on the different views of euthanasia, physicians' strike, advertising in traditional medicine and the principle of beneficence as applied in biomedicine. On euthanasia, physician strike and advertising in traditional medicine, the African traditional view whose birth bed is the African metaphysical conception of "being" and its ontological appurtenances like *unhu*, personality, essence, and *force vitale*, have been emphasized. While honest philosophical reflection may challenge and disrupt many of the beliefs you already hold, it will also enhance and enrich the beliefs you will continue to hold.

While the book advances a more pragmatic view of all the issues considered-euthanasia, physician strike, advertising in traditional medicine and the principle of beneficence- it acknowledges that the answer to the moral problems surrounding majority (if not all) of the issues in biomedicine is very difficult to stipulate in word. As such, the role of judging and deciding problems facing physicians in deciding and judging different cases that arise within the fraternity should not be solely accredited to physicians alone, nor should it be accredited to the government alone. Instead, several parties such as non-governmental organizations, moralists, members of the public, patients/patients committees, physicians, academics and the national government(s) should contribute in the negotiations [of a "just" and rational judgment] of any of the controversial issues in biomedicine before a final deliberation is made.

Introduction

This is a book about euthanasia, physician strikes, advertising in traditional medicine and the principle of beneficence, four of the widely discussed and most contentious issues in medical ethics. The book is intended for scholars and students of philosophy, anthropology, sociology and medicine and anyone else who is interested in issues of biomedicine.

The concepts and definitions of euthanasia, strike, advertising and beneficence have been well documented in the literature, and scholars have provided a number of interpretations to the terms. When looking at different kind of theoretical debates on these biomedical issues held in several academic journals, it is striking how many articles especially from the western world, just arguing for or against any of the issues. Yet, while there is monumental literature on pro-arguments on the one hand and con-arguments on the other, there is patchy literature that examines the nexus between the preservation of medical professionalism through "liberal beliefs and/or practices" and the safeguard of human rights of the ordinary patients, third parties (in patient-physician relations) and the general public with regard to the aforementioned issues. At best, many academics seem to have conceived these constituencies of academic research as irreconcilable research spheres. There is, therefore, need for a more comprehensive research on euthanasia, physician strike, traditional medicine advertising and beneficence especially from Africa where research on these issues have not only been patchy, but very narrowly focused. The latter factor is also true of research by western scholars on these important topics wherein most are limited either to pro- or con-arguments.

In light of this observation, this book conceives as its central argument the need to re-introduce, re-think and re-problematize the moral controversies surrounding euthanasia, physician strike, traditional medicine advertising and the principle of beneficence. This is proposed in an attempt to move beyond the traditional positions by either pro- or con-arguments raised so far to create a more radical holistic and balanced approach that would further develop the field of medical ethics by taking greater account of factors such as liberal life-style, critical questioning, moral intensity and intention development. This is drawn on the realization that the intractable nature of the controversies surrounding the aforementioned issues has been stirred by the threshold question as to whether the issues are morally good or bad. It is in the face of such intellectual moral uneasiness that philosophical inquiry on euthanasia, physician strike, traditional medicine advertising and beneficence begins, hence the present book.

It is acknowledged that the subjects of euthanasia, strike, advertising and beneficence are very broad and far reaching inquiries. In any case, there are a number of strategic hurdles to overcome. The first is that the approach advanced in this book- the liberal, pragmatic and critical questioning approach, of which the moderate view of euthanasia is a product-, is perceived to be foreign to both the African traditional worldview and western philosophy. As such, one may wonder how such a view can gain support in the face of the two warring positions -pro and con-euthanasia, for example- already competing for an answer to the morality of the issues in question. The second concerns the different conceptions of life, its purpose and value the world-over. Is it possible to talk of euthanasia, physician strike, traditional medicine advertising and beneficence in sub-Saharan Africa and still make sense in the debate about the subjects at one hand, and to talk about the same subjects at a global scale on the other hand? The third problem pertains to the geographical epithet "sub-Saharan Africa". Is it possible to develop a broad outline or rather a complete view of euthanasia, physician strike, traditional medicine advertising and beneficence from the perspective of a geographical area, a sub-continent – sub-Saharan Africa- which is only a part of Africa and the world? Wouldn't the contextuality of such a perspective fly into the face of the assumed universality of the ideas of medical ethics, going against the grain of its intersubjective and therefore international use? Or wouldn't this tantamount to lapsing into a kind of truncated conception of euthanasia, strike, advertising and beneficence leaving us with nothing but the narrow vision of local biases, interests and viewpoints? Furthermore, would such a perspective, if it can be circumscribed at all, do justice to a wide range of the lived social experiences of millions of people of Africa who themselves have different cultural histories and circumstances? Perhaps the consoling response to all these questions is the fact that no work can claim to say all that need be said on any subject matter. What is important in any given work is to have a clear vision of what is intended to be achieved. This is not to say that the questions above shall not be fully addressed and examined in this book. In fact, I would like to contend that these questions can be addressed and objections arise overcome if one takes as a starting point that medical issues in Africa, as they are the world over, can never be divorced from people's issues, cultural issues and rational issues. At the same time I would like to draw attention to the fact that general theories, should be related to, if not evaluated from the view point of certain key experiences and questions of people in a particular geographical setting and circumstances. I feel, therefore, persuaded that in this book the highlighted hurdles can be safely handled and overcome.

Much has been said on different aspects of medical ethics, especially from the western world's perspective as scholars tussled with different aspects of the contentious subjects of euthanasia, physician strike, traditional medicine advertising and beneficence in biomedicine. However, it should be noted that western medical ethics are basically a history of individual medical ethicists and physicians whose ideas have been written and preserved on paper. Contrary-wise, African traditional medical ethics do not belong to individual people. Even with the recent publications by prominent African philosophers on African philosophy like John Mbiti, Paulin Hountondji, Tsenay Serequeban, Odera Oruka, among a few others, no written texts especially focusing on African medical ethics in particular have been developed so far; what has been written are works that are mostly dependent on orally transmitted ideas and works that claim to represent African philosophy in general. This in itself makes curious readers to question whether there are no branches of philosophy that can be identified and talked of as is with the case of western philosophy. One thus can raise a crucial question: If Western philosophy has branches such as Metaphysics, Epistemology, Logic, and Ethics/Moral philosophy, Aesthetics, Medical ethics and others, why not African philosophy? Can't we have philosophy branches as African medical ethics or at least African views on medical ethics documented? It is precisely this area: fusing irenicism and intellectual courage that shines through the pages of this work to form a sparkling whole and a wide-ranging survey of biomedical issues that continue to haunt Africa and the global world. This makes this book qualify as a text that seeks to fill in gaps in history to link the past to the present, and speak for the adaptation of African philosophies, reconcile the philosophies with the Western ones and critique them where necessary as a way of refinement not relegation. It is argued in this book that for this to happen, a study of the cultures, particularly the "cultural ideals" of Africa and other "disadvantaged societies" is necessary to bring to light what may be considered the main indices of the "African traditional medical ethics" systems of thought. In other words, culture reflects the people's attitude towards life and the world they live in; it determines what the people consider as fundamental and promotive of their sense of the meaning of human existence.

In this book, historical, hermeneutical and philosophical approaches will be employed in discussing the background of ethics in medicine and the concepts of euthanasia, physician strike, traditional medicine advertising and beneficence. These approaches help making a clear understanding of the etymology, nature and scope of these concepts as issues of great moral concern in medical ethics and in human life in general. Again, the approaches make it feasible to investigate whether the outcome of this study will succeed in engendering the stimulation of moral philosophers, medical professionals and the public especially given the fact that both pro- and con- arguments on the issues considered in this book have failed to provide a philosophically convincing answer to the questions raised around the issues.

This work goes beyond pro- and con- arguments of euthanasia, physician strike, traditional medicine advertising and beneficence to pointing out that cultural philosophy born out of some geographical locations like "African medical ethics" must have certain underlying logic to explain the complexities of the aforementioned issues so as to solve problems confronted by the society from within, and not from without. However, it will be a mark of intellectual philistinism to continue to hold that all Africans conceive reality woof and weft from exactly the same perspective or view point. What Africans have are similar out-looks and spiritual inspiration which enjoy a higher semblance than with views outside the African context. That said, this book makes an attempt to look at the drawing board and see how one can stand with the spate or write-ups on "African medical ethics" and battle with medicine related issues of high moral complexity like euthanasia, physician strike, traditional medicine advertising and beneficence as applied in biomedicine.

Drawing on all these observations, this work contributes to this grey area by demonstrating that the pro- arguments on euthanasia, strike, advertising and beneficence have been extreme, narrowly focused and riddled with "social injustices". On the other hand, the con- arguments such as the obligatory/over-demanding "African traditional view" and those based solely on the Hippocratic Oath and related principles need reconstruction or reconstitution or both; otherwise they cannot be accepted as well on philosophical grounds. As an alternative to pro- and con- views, this work proposes a more pragmatic and liberal view of medical ethics in determining cases of euthanasia, strikes, advertising and beneficence in the medical fraternity. This is achieved through arguments supported with both hypothetical and real "exemplary cases" not only drawn from life experiences of Africans, but of the world at large. The devastating effects and implications drawn from the cases have activated the call for a rethinking and critical questioning of the dormant views of euthanasia, physician strike, traditional medicine advertising and beneficence in biomedicine as a way through which all cases that fall within the precinct of these issues can be judged. This approach (to medical issues) gives advantage to all, that is, the physicians, members of the public and all kinds of patients- the competent and incompetent ones. The virtue of this book, thus, is to ascertain how useful and influential critical questioning is, especially as a strategy through which forces of medical ethics would essentially benefit patients, healthy professionals and the public in general not only in Africa, but in the global world in decision making on historically problematic medical issues. This seems breaking the ground given that no significant amount of energy by scholars in the medical field or ethics in general has been given so far to advance a view as this. Nevertheless, the work acknowledges that the answer to the moral problems such as those pertaining to euthanasia, physician strike, advertising and beneficence in biomedicine is very difficult to stipulate and cannot be epitomized in a word. Thus, even though critical questioning is suggested and advanced in this work, a tricky and difficult question still arises: "Who should be responsible for judging and deciding problematic medical cases such as those to do with euthanasia, strike, advertising and beneficence in biomedicine?" To settle this question, it is argued in this book that the role of judging and deciding problematic medical cases should not be solely accredited to medical doctors. Neither should it be accredited to clients/patients' relatives or patients themselves alone. Instead, several parties which include the patient, moralists, physician(s), patient's relatives, independent organizations, among others should take part in the deliberation of euthanasia cases.

For purposes of thoroughness and clarity, the first three chapters of this book focus on the conception, historical background and clashing views of euthanasia in medical ethics. The fourth chapter looks at the central argument developed in the first three chapters- the proposed "moderate view of euthanasia and the principle of negotiated justice" - and its nexus with democratic civil and individual rights of patients. The fifth, sixth and seventh chapters discuss physicians' strikes, advertising in traditional medicine and the principle of beneficence respectively. The arrangement of chapters, as they are, will enable me to count my successes and failures as I continue in this important philosophical inquiry of offering what I believe will be of great service not only to medical practitioners, but to patients, members of the public and all other interested groups. This intellectual inventory will enable me to question the traditional views of euthanasia, physician strike, traditional medicine advertising and beneficence in biomedicine [pro-and con- arguments] and other such views that for a long time have gone unquestioned. By so doing, the book provides an up-date, invigorates and redirects the debate on burning issues in contemporary medical ethics in Africa and the world-over. The book thus is indeed, more than its predecessors, a thought-provoking representation and demonstration of African philosophers' commitment to reform some approaches in medical fraternity and exhibit a broad outline of medical ethics that African societies and the world at large can adopt for the common good. *Euthanasia and Other Burning Issues in Contemporary Medical Ethics* thus qualifies as food for thought.

Chapter One

Ethics in Medicine: A Philosophical Analysis

Medical ethics like Ethics itself is a branch of practical philosophy. It is a very broad and far reaching inquiry in so far as it has developed from diversified sources and influences. More so, it has many complex moral issues that since time immemorial have troubled the history's finest minds. Given such a background, it would be wise for us to begin with a historical background of Ethics in Medicine; to see how medical ethics as a discipline developed from antiquity to the present. This is what we will consider in the next few pages.

Historical Background of Ethics in Medicine

It is widely believed that good health, of which, health is defined as "a state of complete physical, mental and social well-being and not merely the absence of disease or infirmity"[1] is enjoyed by many if not all people. It is a desire for all. To meet the need and desire of the people to be healthy medicine was therefore obliged to incorporate ethics in all its operations, hence the birth medical ethics.

Before the birth of medical ethics, ethics as a discipline evolved through time. Let us examine how ethics evolved before pursuing further the question on how medical ethics as a discipline came into being and has developed over time.

The history of ethics, that is, about the good, bad, right or wrong has developed under a number of diverse influences and from a variety of sources. Reflection upon ethical matters thus is said to date back to ancient times. Paul Minus notes that:

In the western culture, ethics explicitly began with Plato. Aristotle raised it further to an independent philosophical discipline alongside logic and physics. Its main object was to answer question of the greatest good and the right measures from which rational and virtuous actions would ensue[2].

This connotes that before Plato, ethical issues were only discussed implicitly. Plato and Aristotle raised discussions on ethics to a higher philosophical plane; they made a significant attempt to understand the good and the bad and persuade people to practice the former and avoid the latter. Aristotle, in his *Nicomachean Ethics*, had this to say:

The ultimate purpose of in studying ethics is not as it is in other inquiries, the attainment of theoretical knowledge; we are not conducting this inquiry in order to know what virtue is, but in order to become good, else there would be no advantage in studying it.[3]

What Aristotle is emphasizing here is that ethics is practical in nature; it is a practical philosophy. It studies the values and principles or guidelines by which we must live as well as the goals and justification of these guidelines. In other words, ethics starts with the question: "What is good and why?" This became the central question for ethics since the time of Aristotle.

Contributing to the debate on the nature and origins of ethical principles, Ray Billington asks; "When is it that an ethical principle becomes one such thing?"[4] He looks at the origins of scientific principles and seeks to compare that with ethics. For him, Isaac Newton was the propounder of the principle of gravity in the 17th century. Does this mean that the principle did not exist prior to Newton's utterances? Exporting this to ethics, Billington remarks:

Love thy neighbour as thyself was first written, say, around 1000 BC. Nobody who has read or heard that statement except a psychopath will disagree with it. But did its validity commence only at the time when it was given verbal expression? Of course not! If the principle was universally valid after 1000BC, it was valid even before 1000BC. It was valid from the time homosapien first appeared on this planet and began to interact with members of his species?[5]

Following from Billington's assertion, one can infer that though implicitly, ethics, (which is used interchangeably with morality in this work) has developed over time even in the field of medicine. Tom L. Beauchamp acknowledges this view when he remarks:

In the ancient Western culture, ethics in medicine has been influenced by a religious sect known as Pythagoreanism. Yet, in Medieval Europe, Medical ethics was deeply influenced by Christianity which placed special emphasis on compassion for the ill.[6]

The same view is buttressed by the Biblical injunction: "Thou shalt not kill"[7], which forbids euthanasia. On the same stroke, Tada points out that the medical tradition that has served us so well for more than two thousand years come from Hippocrates and his disciples. These offered to patients care and dignity-important aspects of social life that patients required in order to restore their health. It is this important realization of the Hippocrates that physicians must care for more than the body which gave medical ethics as a discipline the weight and value it enjoys even this day. Since then, the term medical ethics -a term that has enjoyed various usages- has come to mean "the body of thinking and codes of conduct developed by the medical profession"[8] to promote good healthy. This is evident in that "as early as the 16th century B.C, the Hippocratic Oath and *Papyri* documents mentioning priest-physicians with rules laid down on how and when to treat patients already existed."[9] Thus as early as before the 16th century B.C, medical ethics had already become the defining characteristic of a medical profession- a form of professional self-regulatory system. Among other things, the Hippocratic Oath, for example, states: "I will use treatment to help the sick according to my ability and judgment, but I will never use it to injure or wrong the sick."[10] This shows that the Hippocratic Oath has always called physicians to a higher ethical standard to heal, to alleviate suffering/pain and to preserve the sanctity of human life.

In view of the above discussion, it remains crucial to note that the Hippocratic Oath is the most enduring legacy of the practice of medicine, being passed from teacher to students, from old physician to new physician and from generation to generation. The Hippocratic Oath and the tradition surrounding it served mankind well for more than two thousand years and have become the medical ethics and the value system that made medicine the art it has become. The function of the Oath in today's society is the same as when it was first spoken. The Oath calls the physicians to a higher ethical standard than that of the society in general, that

4

is, to do what they could for the patient within the framework of "do no harm but save lives and alleviate suffering". This suggests that the Hippocratic physician forbid euthanasia on moral grounds.

Ethics in medicine having developed through history as has been shown, early contributors on medical issues from ancient Greece like Hippocrates and Pythagoras to medieval and modern age practitioners were all concerned in varying degrees with ethical issues. In one way or another, they saw medicine as a branch of practical reason in which concepts of the good, right and the obligatory were quite central. The 18th century Scottish physician, John Gregory, for instance, begins his treaties on Medical ethics with a definition of medicine that incorporates a clear expression of its moral purpose. He, thus, defines medicine as "the art of preserving health, of prolonging life and of curing diseases."[11] His understanding of medicine is adopted from the Hippocratic Oath. He strongly believes that morality is quite central in medicine. Gregory further argues that physicians should employ virtues such as "sympathy, vigour, patience, compassion, prudence and humanity in dealing with patients so as to feel the misfortunes of fellow creatures."[12] This understanding of the position of ethics in medicine is not only reflected in volumes of professional medical ethics writings but has even reached the status of penetrating into modern medicine with people like James Rachael, Jos Welie, Ten Have, Thomas Sullivan, among others.

It should be remarked, however, that though ethics and medicine are both human oriented activities, the concept "ethics" as it is transposed into medicine has been viewed as a confusing one. This is because people have always disagreed on what is good, bad, right or wrong. Thus the above historical background of the concept "ethics" in medicine has been sketched in order to show that its present day discussion in medical issues like euthanasia, notwithstanding the differences in accent, has significant historical precedent. In fact, the discussion sheds more light on why most of the medical issues, for example, euthanasia have attracted the attention of many scholars and the public throughout the history of Medical ethics.

Conceptual Analysis of Euthanasia

Having shown that ethics can be philosophically examined in line with its historical nexus in medicine, the next task of this work is to discuss the philosophical nature of "euthanasia" as it is one thorn issue in the medical fraternity whose morality has raised the eyebrows of many professional ethicists and the public in general.

Euthanasia

The concept of euthanasia is deeply controversial, for moral as well as practical reasons. It has been a "bone" of contention among moral philosophers, medical ethicists and even the public in general. As a result, the concept has been notoriously understood to the extent that it has received a number of interpretations from different scholars. In general terms, it has been defined as killing, letting die, "mercy killing" and or the most humane intervention possible for patients whose suffering cannot be alleviated through other medical means.[13]

However, besides these generalizations, various attempts to formulate a workable definition of this obscure term have been made. Dyck, for instance, argues that euthanasia originally meant "a painless and happy death."[14] This understanding still appears in the modern literature. The Oxford dictionary, for instance, defines euthanasia as "a gentle and easy death."[15] As can be noted, these definitions are ambiguous. They do not make any reference to whether such death is induced or not. Neither do the definitions clearly state/indicate the person in question (one who would die happily, easily or gently). A definition which tries to do away with these ambiguities has, therefore, come to prevail.

As pointed out by Helga Kuhse, euthanasia now generally means "the bringing about of good death, mercy killing where one person, (A) end the life of another person, (B) for the sake of (B)."[16] She gives an example of a doctor who may disconnect the life support system of an irreversible comatose for the sake of the comatose. Kuhse derives this definition from his analysis of the etymology of the term euthanasia. He notes that the term euthanasia is a compound of two Greek compound words, *eu* –well or good and *thanatos*- death, which literally means "good death."[17] It is good death because it is the end of a patient's pain and suffering. More so, the patient dies through a peaceful and pain free way that is normally administered by a physician. But a critical question can be raised: "What is good death?" It is curious to note that what Kuhse is saying in effect is that the method employed in causing death is painless, though not always, and the act is undertaken solely for the sake of the patient, that is, to end the sufferings of the patient and nothing else. Moreover the person whose life is terminated is presumably hopeless. S/he is getting progressively worse that recovery and or cure cannot be reasonably expected.

It should be emphasized that in the act of euthanasia, termination of life is deliberate, and is done solely for the patient's own good. In this sense, one can loosely understand euthanasia as the termination of a patient's life by another person for the sake of the patient and nothing else. The two features of the act of euthanasia, that is, an act done by another person and for the sake of the patient, are of paramount importance in the discussion of euthanasia. They enable one not to confuse euthanasia with acts of killing like murder, suicide, abortion, infanticide; where for example in the case of abortion, a foetus may be killed for the mother's sake and not for its own sake. Put differently, these two features are eye openers to those who commit themselves to the discussion of euthanasia and its morality. But before paying attention to the morality of euthanasia, let us look at the different types of euthanasia.

Traditional Types of Euthanasia

Euthanasia is found in different forms. Basically, three forms are traditionally known namely; voluntary euthanasia, involuntary euthanasia and non-voluntary euthanasia. I shall look at each in their order.

Voluntary Euthanasia

Voluntary euthanasia has been understood as an act of euthanasia "carried out at the request of the person to whom it is to be applied,"[18] and for the sake of the latter. In other words, euthanasia is voluntary, if the person killed is rational and competent enough to request or give informed consent about a particular action that will lead to his/her death. Thus,

8

voluntary euthanasia is administered at the request of the person killed. Person P, for example, can have his/her life terminated by X at his/her [P] request and for the sake of the latter. The request may be in writing as in the case of a living will or advance directive. In this example, the patient P is competent to request in writing or by advance directive to have his or her life terminated by X [who is normally a physician] when suffering from a distressing and incurable condition, illness or accident have robbed one of all his/her rational faculties such that s/he can no longer able to decide between life and death. Thus if whilst when still competent, the patient expressed the considered wish to die when in a situation such as this, then the person who ends the patient's life in the appropriate circumstances acts upon the patient's request and performs an act of voluntary euthanasia.

Voluntary euthanasia is based on the belief of self-determination and bodily integrity.[19] Brock understands self-determination as meaning "...people's interest in making important decisions about their lives for themselves according to their own values or conceptions of a good life, and in being left free to act on those decisions."[20] Self-determination, so understood, would, therefore, implore us to respect decisions of fully informed and competent patients to refuse life prolonging measures, albeit a miserable one, in favour of a quick death. Thus on the basis of this belief, patients have the right to refuse life-extending medical treatment if they do not see any sense or value in prolonging their misery on earth. Cases of euthanasia arise when because one feels that his/her life is now "miserable," "meaningless" and "hopeless" s/he sees it better requesting death. S/he may be suffering from distressing and incurable disease which causes incessant pain that can no longer be alleviated or is terminally ill such that there is no hope of recovery and cure. For instance, a patient suffering from an incurable disease such as HIV/AIDS knowing that there is no hope of recovery and cure may ask a physician to administer a lethal dose on him so that he dies. He/she may also refuse burdensome medical treatment or demands that medical treatment be stopped, or life support machines be switched off or a person instructs his/her family in advance not to permit the use of artificial life-supporting system, if s/he should become unconscious, or suffers brain damage and being unable to speak for himself/herself or requests that s/he should be given a lethal injection, in the event that s/he suffers third degree burns over most part of his body. Helga Kuhse in the article, *Euthanasia* gives us a clear example of a voluntary euthanasia case:

Mary F. was dying from a progressively debilitating disease. She had reached the stage where she was almost totally paralyzed and periodically, needed a respirator to keep her alive. She was suffering considerable distress. Knowing that there was no hope and that things would get worse, Mary F. wanted to die. She asked her doctor to give her a lethal injection to end her life. After consultation with her family and members of the health care team, Dr H. administered the asked –for lethal injection, and Mary F. died.[21]

This form of euthanasia should be clearly distinguished from physician assisted suicide which occurs when a person who is having difficulties in committing suicide (perhaps because of the seriousness of his illness) without the assistance of another person may ask for the means of suicide

10

like poison or lethal pill to be made available. If the person who wants to kill himself does so using the provided means, then, he has been assisted to commit suicide because the final act is carried out by the very person who is suffering and is feeling that it is "better off dead."[22] It should be emphasized therefore that the final act in voluntary euthanasia is carried out by another person, normally a physician. On the other hand, in physician assisted suicide, the final act is carried out by the very person who wants to die. This is to say that if death is effected by the patient himself, it becomes a suicidal case and not a case of voluntary euthanasia. And, if death is effected by a physician or any other person but without the consent or approval of the patient and or other parties like the patient's relatives among others, the case turns to be murder. It interesting to note that many people prefer physician assisted suicide to voluntary euthanasia because in the former where the patient has to perform the final act himself/herself; there is always more room for the patient to reconsider his position, that is, the desire to die. In other words, it seems possible that a patient who asks for means of suicide like lethal dose to be made available may at the last minute change his mind and not take the dose. Such last minute change of mind cannot possibly be considered in cases of voluntary euthanasia. This is one major reason why it has been argued that assisted suicide is always preferred to voluntary euthanasia.

Involuntary Euthanasia

In instances of involuntary euthanasia, the patient's life is terminated for his own sake against his wishes or views. Or the people or person who kills the patient does not even ask

11

for the consent of the patient to know whether the patient wants to be killed or not. This can be so simply because the patient is no longer competent to make any decision as in cases where one suffers from brain damage or serious brain haemorrhages such that there is no hope of the person recovering. Put differently, the one whose life is terminated even if he is competent is not given room to decide on the fate of his own life. The patient's "will" or views are thus overridden by those of the second or and third parties. Those who initiate the death of the patient normally appeal to the principle of mercy. The principle establishes two component duties; "the duty not to cause further pain or suffering and the duty to end pain or suffering already occurring."[23] This is to say those who effect the death feel that the patient will continually live a "miserable" and "unworthy" life. A case in point is that of a severely injured (beyond cure) and dismembered casualty. This characterization however, is problematic insofar as miserable life and that which makes life worth living may vary. Yet, it should be emphatically reiterated that the bottom line for involuntary euthanasia is that the patient's life is terminated for his or her own sake and nothing else. It is also worth noting that cases of involuntary euthanasia are rare.

Non-voluntary Euthanasia

Euthanasia is non-voluntary when a person whose life is terminated for his or her sake, is not autonomous to choose between life and death herself/himself. The victim who is perhaps demented or mentally retarded is incompetent or too inactive to decide between life and death such that euthanasia is administered without her explicit permission. Brain dead infants, severely handicapped infants, the permanently comatose, Down's Syndromes, hoopla syndrome patients and *sia* twins (twins joined at the back at birth) are some cases in point. Such patients are incompetent and it cannot be surely known whether they want to continue living or not. Of course, one may argue that every human being has a natural inclination to continue living, but it remains a fact that nobody knows for certain whether such persons have interests in life.

It is curious to note that non-voluntary euthanasia is normally initiated by parents, relatives, friends or physicians who feel sorry for the patient or who strongly believe that the patient will live a life so awful that one cannot grasp what it will be like. They would want to satisfy the duty not to cause any further suffering and that of ending pain.

All forms of euthanasia have been looked at. The ensuing paragraphs are therefore devoted to clarify terms; "active euthanasia" and "passive euthanasia" as well as to grapple with the principal question pertaining to the distinction between the two.

Reflection on the Distinction between Active and Passive Euthanasia

It is unwise to attempt to reflect on the distinction between active and passive euthanasia before paying some attention to the concepts "active euthanasia" and "passive euthanasia" themselves. These concepts shall be discussed briefly and separately before looking at the distinction between the two.

Active Euthanasia

This is "the practice of directly bringing about a person's death according to or against that person's wishes."[24] A person who wishes to die, for instance, may request that a lethal injection be administered on him/her or the physician can administer the lethal injection with the request of the patient and such an injection would constitute active euthanasia. This is to say in active euthanasia positive steps to end the life of a patient, typically by lethal injection that is capable of causing the patient to die are well pronounced.

Passive Euthanasia

This type of euthanasia is popularly called *letting die*. It is "the practice of doing nothing to prevent death from occurring."[25] For example, if someone is suffering from an incurable disease, decision may be made not to provide adequate necessary medication to the patient. Or a decision may be made not to treat the patient at all thereby allowing him to die naturally. In fact, a patient is allowed to die by removing from him/her artificial life support systems such as respirators and feeding tubes or simply discontinuing medical treatments necessary to sustain life or letting the patient die by not giving him/her food. Nature thus is simply allowed to take its course resulting in the death of the patient. This is to say that in passive euthanasia or letting die the doctor or family members or whoever is not directly responsible or involved in terminating the life of the patient, though in today's world, one may sue the doctor for negligence.

Now that active and passive euthanasia have been clarified, it should be remarked that the distinction between

14

active and passive euthanasia is thought to be crucial for medical ethics. It is one of the cardinal issues in the euthanasia controversy. More often than not, people disagree on whether there is any morally significant difference between "killing" and "letting a patient die." There is a tug of war amongst philosophers on this question. The idea is that while it is permissible in Medicine, at least in some cases, to withhold treatment and allow a patient to die, it is never permissible on moral grounds to take any direct action designed to kill the patient. In view of this, philosophers like Sullivan and Fletcher have argued that the distinction between active and passive euthanasia is morally relevant. Fletcher for instance, argues that "one can make a sharp distinction one that will stand up in law between 'permitting to die' and 'causing' death."[26] He makes reference to Jewish and Christian tradition particularly, Roman Catholic thought. This line of thinking describes passive euthanasia as a failure to use 'extraordinary means' or employ unusual treatment like respirators, organ transplantation among others, hence permitting the patient to die; and active euthanasia as failure to use or provide standard care- "ordinary means" such as antibiotics hence causing death of the patient. Thus whilst passive euthanasia can be described as failure to use extraordinary means hence allowing the patient to die, active euthanasia can be described as failure to use the "ordinary means" hence causing the death of the patient. This is to say that for Fletcher, passive euthanasia is indirect but active euthanasia involves direct intervention to bring about the death of the patient. In other words, the latter – "ordinary means" of causing death of the patient can be characterized as "killing" or "causing death" whilst the former can be characterized as "permitting to die". Fletcher, in a bid to shed more light on the issue under consideration further argues that "a distinction between active and passive euthanasia can be more clarified if we draw a distinction between a drug administered to cause death and a drug administered to ease pain which has the added effect of shortening life."[27] This doctrine seems to be accepted by some doctors. It is, for instance, endorsed in a statement adopted by the House of Delegates of the America Medical Association (AMA) on December 4, 1973:

> ...the causation of the employment of extraordinary means to prolong the life of the body when there is irrefutable evidence that biological death is imminent is the decision of the patient and or his immediate family. The advice and judgment of the physician should be freely available to the patient and or his immediate family.[28]

However, two prime questions which appear to be more or less the same can be raised against the doctrine: "Why is the distinction important and of any moral relevance if both instances; permitting to die and causing death have the same effect of shortening life? And, is it a failure to achieve the goal of medicine; that of preserving health, curing diseases and prolonging life of one who is ill?"

The questions raised clearly show that a strong case can be made against the distinction between active euthanasia and passive euthanasia. I would support Rachels in arguing that the notion that there is morally significant difference between active and passive euthanasia is wrong. Rachels makes it clear that "one reason why so many people think that there is an important moral difference between active and passive euthanasia is that they think killing someone is morally worse than letting someone die."[29] This is to say that there is no moral difference between active and passive euthanasia except in semantic terms. To reinforce this contention, Rachels invites us to consider two cases exactly alike except for one reason that one involves killing whereas the other involves letting someone die. In case one:

Smith stands to gain a large inheritance if anything should happen to his six-year old cousin. One evening while the child is taking his bath, Smith sneaks into the bath and drowns the child, and then arranges things so that it will look like an accident. In the second case, Jones also stands to gain if anything should happen to his six-year old cousin. Like Smith, Jones sneaks in planning to drown the child in his bath. However, just as he enters the bathroom Jones sees the child slip and hit his head and fall down in the water. The child drowns all by himself 'accidentally' as Jones watches and does nothing.[30]

Now who is morally better between Smith and Jones? It is at this point that all those who support Fletcher and Sullivan are urged to reconsider their views on this matter. In fact, it seems clear that the only difference between the two cases is that Smith killed the child whereas Jones 'merely' led the child die. But surely either man did not behave better from a moral point of view since they had the same intention. As Rachels argues, if the difference between killing and letting die were in itself a morally important matter, one should say that Jones' behaviour was less reprehensible than Smith's. But analysing carefully the cases under view, this would be a haste generation. It should be reiterated that, in the first place, both men acted from the same motive, personal gain and both had exactly the same end-in-view when they acted. Thus those who argue that Jones does nothing miss the point. It should be brought to light that Jones indeed does something- he lets the child die in much the same way "one may insult another by way of not shaking his hand."[31]

On the same note, in passive euthanasia as in cases of active euthanasia, the doctor does something that result in the death of another; not providing medication to the patient. This connotes that passive euthanasia like active euthanasia, for any purpose of moral assessment, is a type of action nonetheless. This is probably one other reason why both forms of euthanasia are considered morally wrong in most if not all African countries. In Mozambique, Malawi and Zimbabwe for example, both forms of euthanasia carry a jail sentence and are considered morally wrong. They (active and passive euthanasia) have no practical and moral difference and so they are both condemned morally. Supporting the same strand of thought, Wankler argues that:

> The distinction between active and passive euthanasia has no moral relevance since what is of significance for morality is moral responsibility for death. If intentions, measures and outcomes are the same between killing and permitting death to occur, then, it cannot make any oral difference as to what form of causal instrument is involved in bringing about death. Thus if doctors who carry out euthanasia, either passive or active, have the same intention of bringing about death, then, it means that from a moral point of view both doctors are equally responsible for their actions. They are in the same moral position.[32]

18

Considered from this angle, the distinction between active and passive euthanasia is therefore theoretical and of no moral significance. In a nutshell, the preceding explications stand to concretize the major premise that those who argue for or against any instance of euthanasia merely because it is either active or passive make a conceptual mistake. They need to reconsider their positions. Yet, one important question can still be raised: "Does euthanasia morally help or it too often simply adds to one evil still another?" This is the question this work shall grapple with in the ensuing paragraphs.

Notes

1. Gilbert Lawrence, "Medical ethics" in Vicenio V, (Ed), *Doing Ethics in Context*, Orbis Books, New York, 1994, p. 162.

2. Paul M. Minus, (Ed) (1993), *The Ethics of Business in Global Economy*, Kluwer Academic Publishers, Ohio, p.23.

3. See Boss, J.A. *Perspectives on Ethics*, Mayfield Publishing Company, California, 1997, p. 1.

4. Ray Billington, *Philosophy: An introduction to Moral thought*, Routledge & Kegan Paul ltd, London, 1993, p.31.

5. Ray Billington, 1993, p.31.

6. Tom L. Beauchamp, (Ed), Medical *Ethics; The moral responsibilities of Physicians*, Prentice Hall, New Jersey, 1984, p.12.

7. Exodus 20 v.13, *The Holly Bible, New International Version*, International Bible Society, Colorado, USA, 1984.

8. Gilbert Lawrence, 'Medical Ethics' in Vicenio V, (Ed), *Doing Ethics in Context*, Orbis Books, New York p. 162.

9. Gilbert Lawrence, 1994, p. 162.

10. Jones, W.H.S.(Trans)., *Hippocrates* 'Selections from the Hippocratic Corpus' in Veatch, R. (Ed), *Cross Cultural Perspectives in Medical Ethics*, J & Burllett Publishers, Boston, 1989, p.29.

11. Tom L. Beauchamp, (Ed), 1984, p.31.

12. Tom L. Beauchamp, (Ed), 1984, p.34.

13. West, L. J. "Reflections on the Right to Die". In Lennars, A.A. ed. *Sociology: Essays in Honor of Edwin S. Shneidman.* Jason Aronson Inc: London, 1993, p. 359-376.

14. Dyck, J.A., "An alternative to the ethic of euthanasia" in Arthur, J. (Ed). *Morality and moral controversies*, 3rd ed, Prentice Hall, 1981, p.159.

15. Bucherfield, R.W., *The Oxford English Dictionary*, vol v, Clarendon Press, Oxford, 1989, p.444.

16. Helga Kuhse, "Euthanasia" in Singer, P. *A Companion to Ethics*, Basil Blackwell, Oxford, 1991.

17. Helga Kuhse, 1991.

18. Helga Kuhse, 1991.

19. West, L. J. "Reflections on the Right to Die". In Lennars, A.A. ed. Sociology: Essays in Honor of Edwin S. Shneidman. Jason Aronson Inc: London, 1993, p. 359-376.

20. Brock, D.W. "Voluntary Active Euthanasia" In: Arras, J.D & Steinbock, B. eds. Ethical Issues in Modern Medicine. Mayfield Publishing Company: London, 1995, p. 295-309.

21. Helga Kuhse, 1991.p.129.

22. Kuhse, H. "Euthanasia" in Peter Singer, *A Companion to Ethics*, Basil Blackwell, Oxford, 1991, 1979, p.128.

23. Jonathan Glover, *Causing Death and Saving Lives*, Wadsworth, Penguin, 1987, p.183.

24. McDonald, M.J. *Contemporary Moral Issues in a Diverse Society*, Wadsworth Publishing Company, 1981, p.160.

25. Larry, May (Ed). *Applied Ethics; A multicultural Approach*, Prentice Hall, New Jersey, 1994, p.488.

26. Fletcher, G. P. in Arthur, J. (Ed), *Morality and Moral Controversies*, 3rd ed, Prentice Hall, New Jersey, 1981, p.150.

27. Fletcher, G. P. in Arthur, J. (Ed), 1981, p.150.

28. Fletcher, G. P. in Arthur, J. (Ed), 1981, p.150.

29. Rachael, J. "Active and Passive Euthanasia" in *The New England Journal of Medicine*, vol.292, 1975, p. 78-80.

30. Rachael, J. vol.292, 1975, p. 78-80.

31. Rachael, J. vol.292, 1975, p. 78-80.

32. Wankler, E. "Is the Killing/ letting Die Distinction Normatively Neutral?" in *Canadian Philosophical Review: Dialogue*, Volume xxx, no3, summer/ e'te, 1991, p. 309-312.

Chapter Two

Clashing Views on Euthanasia

Having paid attention to the concepts "ethics" and "euthanasia" separately, let us examine how and why the morality of the latter is a subject of debate. Arguments for and against euthanasia will therefore be presented in a bid to show how the morality of euthanasia is a contested notion and, why it does need incisive intellectual investigation.

Pro- euthanasia Arguments

The morality of euthanasia has an understanding which is very porous. There is no consensus amongst those who labour themselves to reflect on the morality of euthanasia. Consequently, two schools of thought have cropped in, making the morality of euthanasia even more complex, obscure and difficult to philosophically unpack.

Among versions emanating from the debate on the morality of euthanasia, two intriguing and very different counterweights, which seem fundamentally significant, have taken the toll. One is summed up in the view of Fredrick Stenn, Margaret Battin and Carl Becker. These scholars have defended euthanasia on moral, religions and rational grounds. Generally, their views claim that euthanasia is morally right. It is a fundamental right of anyone wishes to have his or her life terminated, and to deny one who wants his life terminated is inhumane and unjust. Thus, it is out of this simple logic that euthanasia is considered as inherently morally right.

One of the prominent advocates of euthanasia, Stenn has employed a principle of autonomy in reinforcing his argument. The word "autonomy" is a legacy from ancient Greece. It is derived from the Greek compound "*autos* (self) and *nomos* (rule or law) first combined to refer to self-governance in the Greek city- states"[1] where citizens were given the mandate to formulate their own laws. The most general idea of personal autonomy in moral philosophy is self –governance; forming one's own self by adequate knowledge and understanding; free from controlling interference by others, government or personal limitations. The general idea of autonomy is linked in philosophical literature to several allied concepts such as the freedom to choose, the creation of a personal moral position and accepting responsibility for one's actions. The principle of autonomy, in fact, requires that "we regard others as rightfully self-governing in matters of their choice and action…"[2] In other words, the principle of autonomy contends that values and beliefs of the patient should be the primary moral consideration in determining what is to be done to the patient or in deciding the fate of the patient. In the light of this principle, Stenn argues "…man chooses how to live, let him choose how to die. Let man choose when to depart, where and under what circumstances the harsh winds that blow over the terminus of life must be subdued."[3] Stenn's position shows that the main thrust of his philosophical argument lies in the principles of autonomy. It springs from the assumption that all individuals, whether young or old, are in a position to ascertain their own interests either verbally or otherwise more competently than anyone else. For instance, if an elderly competent patient declares that he wants life support systems to be removed because he does not value prolonged life, then, he should have life supporting systems removed even if family members might object. Expressed differently, the principle of autonomy contends that the patient's values and values should be the basis for determining what is in his or her best interests. This is to say that, for Stenn, euthanasia is a fundamental moral right of anyone who wishes to have his/her life terminated. In short, Stenn is of the view that it is morally right to terminate the patient's life if the patient requests this on the moral grounds of autonomy.

Margaret Battin has also supported this line of thought. She argues that physician-assisted suicide should be allowed. Battin seems to be considering physician-assisted suicide as a form of euthanasia (despite the distinction between physician-assisted suicide and euthanasia as shown in the preceding paragraphs). Battin thus argues that "various forms of euthanasia are taking root in some cultures, for instance, active euthanasia has been practiced without major difficulties in Netherlands. In Germany assisted suicide is allowed; why not in America?"[4] It is against this background that Battin argues that even though passive euthanasia in the form of withdrawal or withholding of treatment is common in United States, still, more forms of euthanasia such as the physician – assisted suicide should be allowed. She adds that "physician assisted suicide has the advantage of giving the patient a greater range of autonomy and of keeping things under a physician's control, especially for those who are severely ill."[5] All what Battin (though seems to be misunderstanding assisted suicide as a form of euthanasia) is that more forms of euthanasia in the form of withdrawal or withholding treatment should be allowed morally in the United States and even in other states.

In line with the above contention, Becker argues that all forms of active euthanasia are morally right. He explores Buddhist view of death and suicide and attempts to apply

25

these ideas to recent debates about euthanasia. Like Hobbes who asserts that "one ought to serve his own interests because he can do nothing else,"[6] Becker advocates psychological egoism. He enters the debate from a Buddhist perspective which unlike the Western one, does not regard death as an evil or as something to be avoided. Traditionally, Buddhism "does not view death as a bad thing or even as an ending. Rather, death is a transition from one stage of life to another. For this reason, euthanasia is not condemned as long as a person had placed himself or herself in the right state of mind"[7] that is, being physically, spiritually and rationally prepared to die. It is from this background that Becker argues that it is inhumane and morally unjustifiable to keep someone alive who is physically, spiritually and rationally prepared to die and indeed wants to die. He thus further argues that "a key to this is that a person accepts responsibility for his or her own life choices. When euthanasia is prohibited, it means that 'a person is deprived of the final act of taking responsibility for his or her own life'"[8]. What Becker is contending is that, the person who wants his or her life terminated should be mentally, spiritually and rationally prepared to die. S/he should not be forced to terminate his or her own life but should do so out of will and self-determination.

It is curious to note that Becker seems to be employing two principles of medical ethics namely, the principle of autonomy and the principle of mercy. The former has been discussed in the preceding paragraphs. The latter principle establishes two component duties-"the duty to act to end pain or suffering already occurring and the duty not to cause further pain or suffering."[9] It should be emphasized that these duties are to be satisfied merely for the sake of the patient. This connotes that, for Becker, if the patient suffering from an incurable disease is experiencing incessant severe pain that can no longer be alleviated requests to have his or her life terminated, permission on the basis of the principle of mercy should be granted. To deny euthanasia to such a patient is to violate the medical principle of mercy, Becker would argue.

Pro-euthanasia arguments have been presented. Let us now turn to con-euthanasia arguments. This will enable us to compare the two positions and examine whether either of the positions is worth pursuing.

Con- euthanasia Arguments

The underlying argument for pro-euthanasia partisans is that euthanasia is morally wrong. Besides, it is not a moral right since every human being has a right to life. Prominent among the critics who set forth to dispel the arguments for the morality of euthanasia include Thomas Aquinas, William Gay, Henk Ten Have and Jos Welie, among others.

Against the claim that euthanasia is morally right, Aquinas for instance, argues that "everything naturally loves itself and, every part as such belongs to the whole. Now every man is part of the community and so, as such belongs to the community. Thus, having his life terminated injures himself and the community"[10] to which he belongs.

What Aquinas is contending is that euthanasia since it involves termination of life by other individual(s) violates the community to which the one whose life is terminated is a member. For these reasons, Aquinas would conclude that euthanasia is morally wrong.

It seems clear that though Aquinas' view is contentious, it has gained wide acceptance and veneration through ages especially due to its respect for sanctity of life and conformity to "Biblical Ethics" which is commonly taken as the foundation for the whole of the ethics. In other words, Aquinas' position has been perceived considerably significant in that it has some affinity with the Biblical rule; "Do not kill."[11] The prohibition suggests that human life is too sacred to be tampered with or to be entrusted to human control. Human beings are therefore barred from terminating other people's lives. To this effect, anyone who terminates another person's life commits a crime against the dignity that belongs to that person as a human being. More so, s/he sins against God who gives life.

In line with the above, Fletcher has forwarded a consequentiality argument against the morality of euthanasia. His argument can be called "the argument from practical effects". He argues that "sometimes the euthanasiasts (those who perform the final act) commit suicide thus, making two deaths instead of one. Sometimes they are tried for murder in courts of law."[12] This is to say that euthanasia has consequential effects, both social and psychological, which are "nauseating" to contemplate. Thus, Fletcher is of the view that euthanasia is morally wrong.

Williams contributing to the debate on euthanasia forwards four arguments against the morality of euthanasia. His first argument is drawn from his understanding of human nature; an argument from nature. He argues that:

Every human being has a natural inclination to continue living. Our reflexes and responses fit us to fight attackers, flee wild animals and dodge out of the way of trucks. In our daily lives, we exercise the caution and care necessary to protect ourselves. Our psychological bodies are

28

similarly structured for survival right down to the molecular level. When we are cut, our capillaries seal shut, our blood clots and fibrinogen is produced to start the process of healing the wound. When we are invaded by bacteria, antibodies are produced to fight against the alien organisms, and their remains are swept out of the body by special cells designed for cleaning up work.[13]

What William is driving home is that the inclination towards living indicates that euthanasia does violence to the natural goal of survival. It is literally acting against nature because all the processes of human nature are bent towards the end of bodily survival and not natural death. In this sense, death on request or imposed on a patient by another, even in those cases where death seems to be inevitable, is contradictory to human nature. William's argument can be understood through simple logic presented below:

Premise1: All processes of human nature such as reflexes and responses bent towards the natural goal of bodily survival.

Premise2: Anything that violates the natural goal of bodily survival is morally wrong.

Premise3: Euthanasia does violence to the natural goal of survival.

Conclusion: Therefore, euthanasia is morally wrong. It is thus out of this argument that Williams' analysis of the morality of euthanasia can pass the logic of reason.

Williams' second argument against euthanasia is more akin to the one just discussed above. It is an argument from self-interest. He argues that "the natural will and interest to live is strong in all of us. And anything that weakens our

29

determination by suggesting that there is an easy way out is ultimately against our own interest."[14] More so, Williams argues that "our contemporary medicine does not possess perfect and complete knowledge. A mistaken diagnosis is possible and, so is a mistaken prognosis."[15] This implies that we may believe that we are dying of a disease when, as a matter of fact, we may not be. We may think that we have no hope of recovery when, as a matter of fact, our chances are quite good. In such circumstances, if euthanasia were permitted we would die needlessly and prematurely. This means that since euthanasia contains in it the possibility that we will work against our own interest if we practice it or allow it to be practiced on us, it is morally wrong.

The third argument employed by Williams is teleological. Though drawn from practical effects of euthanasia (like Fletcher's presented before) Williams argues from another angle. In his argument, Williams concedes that "doctors and nurses are, for the most part, totally committed to saving lives. A life lost is, for them, almost a personal failure, an insult to their skills and knowledge."[16] Besides, Williams argues:

> Euthanasia as a practice has a corrupting influence such that in any case that is severe, doctors and nurses might not try hard enough to save patients. They might decide that the patient would simply be better off dead and take the steps necessary to make sure that death comes about.[17]

An analysis of this argument reveals that the attitude created by allowing euthanasia may result in the overall decline in the quality of medical care. It also creates a sense of distrust and fear in patients. They (patients) may worry that any form of euthanasia can be imposed on them by health care professionals without their consent or even the consent of their immediate relatives. Williams thus concludes that euthanasia is morally wrong.

The final argument that Williams forwards to discredit the morality of euthanasia is more or less the same as the one presented in the previous discussion. He calls it a "slippery slope argument". A slippery slope argument can be defined as an argument which shows that a tricky situation may be allows to prevail not because it is the most desirable one but due to lack of clarity and consensus over it. And, once the situation is allowed to take root, it becomes extremely difficult to stop or control or stop. Williams, thus, argues that if people relax the prohibitions of killing and allow euthanasia, this would lead to the killing of innocent people. He remarks:

If a person apparently hopelessly ill may be allowed to take his own life, then, he may be permitted to deputies others to do it for him should he no longer be able to act. The judgment of others then becomes a ruling factor. Already at this point, euthanasia is not personal and voluntary for others are acting on behalf of the patient as they see it fit. This may well incline them to act on behalf of other patients who have not authorized them to exercise their judgment.[18]

As previously highlighted, this denotes that euthanasia is prone to abuse and so can lead to appalling increase of crimes such as infanticide, geronticide and genocide, among others. Those looking after the patient might terminate the patient's life if they feel it necessary and not because death has been requested. They can do so out of hatred, boredom or and in order to inherit patient's property. A case in point is that of the Nazi Germany where Germans eliminated a great number of Jews (who fell ill and visited hospital) out of hatred and or racism in the name of involuntary euthanasia, a practice that was also known as anti-Semitism or as eugenics. All this concretize the fact that euthanasia may be abused and result in genocide. Hence, euthanasia is morally wrong, Williams would argue. The Zimbabwean people, among other Africans are also against euthanasia. Let us look at their position from an African view as Zimbabweans are Africans and their voice can be used to represent Africa.

African Traditional View of Euthanasia

The African traditional culture is one perspective that abnegates the morality of euthanasia. This is to say that though treated separately in this book the African view of euthanasia falls under con-euthanasia arguments.

In this book, we shall use the term Africa to refer to the sub-Saharan Africa and not the entire continent of Africa. The African view of euthanasia possibly springs from the understanding of personhood by Africans. In the next few paragraphs we shall therefore briefly articulate the conception of personhood in the African traditional thought before critiquing the African view of euthanasia. This account would help us to show how the people of Africa's beliefs influence the law and medical ethics in the region on euthanasia issue.

It is paramount to begin our discussion on African traditional view of euthanasia by pointing to a major and significant contrast between the African conception of personhood and the conception found in the western thought. As rightly acknowledged by Menkiti the major contrast worth noting is that "most western views of man abstract this or that feature of the lone individual and then proceed to make it the defining or essential characteristic which entities aspiring to the description 'man' must have."[19] For example, Descartes in defining what he himself is employs the phrase *"cogito ergo sum'* which literally means, 'I think, therefore, I am"[20] for nothing can think unless it is something. This serves to mean that, for Descartes, the defining and key aspect of personhood is the "cogito"- the thinking self- which wills, imagines, doubts and thinks and, not the physical body. He further emphasizes that the 'cogito' is clear, distinct, independent and known by itself.

Contrary to the above stated view, the African scholars surveyed, with the possible exception of Ghanaian philosopher Kwame Gyekye, regard African concepts of the individual and self to be almost totally dependent on and subordinate to social entities and cultural processes.[21] Generally, the African traditional view of man denies that persons can be defined by focusing on this or that physical or psychological characteristics of the lone individual. Rather, persons are defined by reference to the environing community. This idea has been put forward by several African philosophers. Kenyan theology professor John S. Mbiti, for example, believes that the individual has little latitude for self-determination outside the context of the traditional African family and community. He writes:

Whatever happens to the individual happens to the whole group, and whatever happens to the whole group happens to the individual'. The individual can only say: 'I am, because we are; and since we are, therefore I am'; this is a cardinal point in the understanding of the African view of personhood.[22]

Concurring with Mbiti, South African philosophy professor Augustine Shutte, cites the Xhosa proverb: *umuntu ngumuntu ngabantu* (a person is a person through persons).[23] He elaborates that: This (proverb) is the Xhosa expression of a notion that is common to all African languages and traditional cultures.[24] It cuts across all African cultures. In the same stroke, Achebe commenting on Africa and Africans noted that Africa is not only a geographical expression; it is also a metaphysical landscape-it is in fact a view of the world and of the whole cosmos perceived from a particular position. Achebe goes further to argue that being an African is more than just a matter of passports or of individual volition[25] but of sensibility and responsibility. For Achebe and convincingly so being an African carries penalties. Okot P'Bitek[26] picks up this argument and stresses that in African philosophy, man is not born free to do whatever he wants; in fact it is not even desirable to be so even if it were possible. Thus persons are defined by reference to the environing community, not by focusing on this or that physical or psychological characteristics of the lone individual. One obvious conclusion to be drawn from all these African scholars' view of personhood is that, as far as Africans are concerned, the reality of the communal world takes precedence over the reality of individual life histories, whatever these may be. Put differently, personhood is defined by reference to other members of the same community. In this view, physicians in the African context for example are defined through members of their society (the patients and the public in general). They are physicians because of the people (patients and members of the public) they serve and are part. The relationship between physicians and other members of his/her community (patients and members of the public) can be represented by the syllogism:

1) An individual in the African society is defined through others;
2) A physician (in the African view point) is an individual who lives in a society. Therefore, a physician is defined through other members of his/her society.

As already spelled out the reality of the communal world takes precedence over the reality of individual life histories, whatever these may be. In the light of this, it is inescapably true that in the African context and indeed other contexts where people share the same idea of personhood and communal life, allowing euthanasia is violation of the public trust- a complete failure to exhibit the prime duty and responsibility-of serving and preserving lives- to other members of their community. It is thus not only morally unjustifiable but also unfair and unjust to other members of the community. This is so because in any society (where people have the common goals) each member has his duties and responsibilities which s/he should accomplish with all the cogency, dedication and efficiency for his good and the good of the society. This is what Achebe stresses when he says "an African is born with duties and responsibility to his society and the society in turn bestows rights and privileges on its members."[27] The values of individuals and individual rights, for example, are normally overridden by the values and rights of the community as a whole (to which the individual belongs). This justifies the African traditional view of euthanasia which strictly disallows any form of euthanasia to be executed by physicians, member(s) of the public or anyone who deems it necessary.

Of course, Gyekye though an African supports moderate or restricted communalism, which contends that African view of personhood accommodates, besides communal values, values of individuality, social commitments and self-attention. He argues:

> Though in its basic trust and concerns, African view of personhood gives prominence to duties toward the community and its members, it does not do so to the detriment of individual rights whose existence and value it recognizes or should recognize.[28]

However, it should be noted that what Gyekye says (basing on his research of personhood in the Akan people of Ghana) is only true in principle as in most traditional African ethnic groups, for example, the SiSwati of Swaziland, the Shona/Ndebele of Zimbabwe, the Mandau/Shangani of Mozambique, the Zulus of South Africa, the Tswana of Botswana, the Chewa of Malawi and the Swahili of Tanzania (ethnic groups I am well conversant with) the values of individuals, individual rights for instance, are normally overridden by the values of the community as a whole simply because an individual is considered a person through other persons/members of the same community.

Let us consider in some detail one example of an ethnic group, the Shona, which embraces the aforementioned African view of personhood for us to understand better the African traditional view of euthanasia. In Shona traditional culture as has been seen with the Zulu and of course other African cultures, *munhu munhu kubudikidza navamwe* (*lit* a person is a person through others meaning a person is defined by reference to the society in which s/he is part). There is indispensable interdependence between members of the same community. This interdependence justifies the existence of persons in that community. This is to say that in the Shona culture as with other African cultures, if an individual is to exist as a full person, there should be a community to which the person belongs or is part. And, for a community to exist there should be individual persons belonging to it. In other words, there is a symbiotic relationship between a person and the community to which the person belongs. Neither the community nor the person can exist without implying, the other explicitly or implicitly. To this effect, a person in the aforementioned culture should conform to certain customs and values which guarantee societal solidarity, unity, peace and harmony if s/he is to be recognized as a full person. Failure to conform to these standards denigrates and devalues his or her personhood. And normally, persons of the "sort" are given pejorative or diminutive names like *Zibhinya* (murderer), *Zibenzi* (a fool) and *Zimbwa* (a dog mannered person). All these names have a prefix *Zi-* which in Shona is derogative and means the referred is no longer recognized as a member of the realm of persons. S/he has lost ties with the community to which s/he is belonged. This implies that every member is obliged to observe and cherish certain values in the culture, of course, not forgetting their own individual values in their conduct with other members of the community if they (individuals) are to be recognized as full persons. Otherwise, the individuals risk losing their personhood as personhood is something that is acquired and not something which results merely from the fact that one is born from "human seed."

To foster and safeguard personhood, the Shona culture strives to preserve the lives of its members and all other societal values/belief systems. For instance, there are health facilities and health professionals – the traditional healers who commit themselves to cure diseases, to preserve health and prolong lives of the members of their communities. Life thus is the most highly sacred and regarded societal gift in the Shona culture as in other African cultures. As such, death is considered as the most serious and severe loss of the community. And if the death was initiated by another individual in the community, the culprit faces the wrath of the law. The culprit is considered a murderer, a witch, an outcast or retrogressive element in the society and is liable for severe punishment. Besides, there is witch-hunt among Shona, for example; a practice which is meant to safeguard and guarantee human life. Other members of the community also mourn over the death or injury of a fellow member. Of course, these people believe that there is a spiritual world where ancestors reside and where one finds place when s/he "departs". But as seen, the bodily life is also of great value. Actually, the duality of personhood-both the physical and metaphysical parts of personhood are of considerable values. And so, it is believed that if one's bodily life is terminated by another, the wrathful vengeance of the avenging spirit-*"ngozi"* which can only be pacified by reparation causes unfathomable sorrow on the murderer and his or her family. As acknowledged by Father Emanuel Ribeiro in his novel *Muchadura*- "You shall confess", the wrath of the avenging spirit would work havoc, for example, cause series of inexplicable deaths, diseases and unaccountable is fortunes

38

upon the family of the murderer[29]. As such, the life of a person is something sacrosanct and reverential. No one should take it upon himself or herself to end another person's life whether on personal grounds or through the "law". It is for these reasons among others that the Shona and by extension Africans abnegate euthanasia on whatever grounds. They consider euthanasia as a practice that is inherently morally wrong;-a practice that harms the whole community and, which also threatens the posterity and perpetuation of the community. In short, the Shona and indeed most if not all African cultures euthanasia is a public matter insofar as it involves our conception of how we ought to live together in an ideal society. Death on request or imposed on others-euthanasia- is therefore considered a crime against the dignity of the victim and the community in which the victim (patient) is part. It is against the group's ethics. To this end, the African view has also penetrated into the African medical fraternity such that euthanasia is considered wrong from a moral point of view of the African people.

Notes

1. Wankler, E., 'Is the Killing/ letting Die Distinction Normatively Neutral?' in *Canadian Philosophical Review: Dialogue*, Volume xxx, no3, summer/ e'te, 1991, p. 309-312.

2. James Rachael, 'Active and Passive Euthanasia' in *The New England Journal of Medicine*, vol.292, 1975, p. 44.

3. Stenn, F., "A plea for Voluntary Euthanasia" in *New England Journal of Medicine*, vol. 303, 9 October, 1980, p.891.

4. Margaret Battin, "Euthanasia" in Deveer, D.V and Regan (Ed)., *Health Care : An introduction,* Temple University Press, USA, 1987.

5. Margaret Battin, "Euthanasia" in Deveer, D.V and Regan (Ed), 1987.

6. Margaret Battin, "Euthanasia" in Deveer, D.V and Regan (Ed), 1987.

7. Dewey, R.E.(Ed)., *An introduction to Ethics,* Macmillan Publishing Company, New York, 1999, p.32.

8. Carl B. Becker, 'Buddhist views of suicide and Euthanasia' in May, L. (Ed). *Applied Ethics: A multicultural Approach,* Prentice Hall, New Jersey, 1994, p.517.

9. Carl B. Becker, 1994, p.517.

10. Dewey, R.E. (Ed), 1999, p.159.

11. Deuteronomy xxx 11:39 in *The Holly Bible,* International Bible Society, USA, 1984.

12. Williams, G.J, 'The wrongness of euthanasia' in White, J.E., *Contemporary moral problems,* 5th Ed, West publishing company, USA, 1991, P.195.

13. Fletcher, J., "Euthanasia; Our Right to Die" in Clark R., *Introduction to moral reasoning,* West publishing company, New York, 1986, p.192.

14. Williams, G.J. 1991, p.195.

15. Williams, G.J. 1991, p.196.

16. Williams, G.J. 1991, p.196.

17. Williams, G.J. 1991, p.196.

18. Williams, G.J. 1991, p.196.

19. Menkiti, I. A. "Person and Community in African Traditional Thought" in Wright, R.A. (Ed)., *African Philosophy, An Introduction,* 3rd Ed, University press of America, New York, 1984, p.171.

20. Descartes, R. "Meditations on first Philosophy" in *A Companion of Philosophy*, Cambridge Press, 1986, p.312.

21. Gyekye K. *The Unexamined Life: Philosophy and the African Experience*, Accra. Ghana Universities Press, 1988: 31-32

22. Mbiti, J, *African Religion and Philosophy*, Heinemann, London, 1969, p.113.

23. Augustine Shutte, Philosophy for Africa, South Africa. University of Cape Town Press, 1993: 46-47

24. Augustine Shutte, Philosophy for Africa, South Africa. University of Cape Town Press, 1993: 46-47

25. Achebe C, Hopes and Impediments, New York. Anchor Books, 1990:17

26. Okot P'Bitek, in Wiredu K. *A Critique of Western Scholarship on African Religion*, Wiley-Blackwell,

    2005

27. Chinua Achebe, *Hopes and Impediments*, New York. Anchor Books, 1990:17

28. Kwame Gyekye, "Person and Community in African Thought" in Roux A.P.J.(Ed)., *The African Philosophy Reader*, Routledge, London, 1992,p.334

29. Father Emanuel Ribeiro, *Muchadura*, Mambo Press, Gweru, 1968.

Chapter Three

Critical Assessment of Views on Euthanasia

As has been seen in the previous discussion, both pro-euthanasia and con-euthanasia arguments seem to be equally convincing. However, the truth is, both positions cannot be right at the same time. Either of the positions or both are wrong. It is in light of this observation that I propose the need to subject both pro-euthanasia and con-euthanasia arguments under scrutiny before challenging them.

A Critical Analysis of Pro-euthanasia Arguments

Philosophical arguments for euthanasia have been presented in the prior discussion. They however seem to be convincing yet fail to provide a conclusive answer to the question of the morality of euthanasia. Pro-euthanasia arguments particularly, the argument from autonomy, for example, shows that the principle is a prima facie obligation and not an absolute one. A prima facie principle is "that principle always to be acted upon unless it conflicts on a particular occasion with an equal or stronger principle."[1] A prima facie principle, we might say, is always right and binding all other things being equal. It can only be overridden in those circumstances when it conflict with equal or stronger obligation(s).

It is in this light that autonomy as a prima facie is problematic. It cannot help us much in the judging of conflicting principles. It can be overridden, for instance, when it conflicts with medicine's duty to preserve health and prolong life especially in those cases when a patient who is experiencing short lived pain requests that euthanasia be applied on him. In this case, the patient's choice is overridden (though not everywhere) by consideration of medicine's duty to preserve health and prolong life by curing diseases. The principle does not also apply to some individual, for instance, the comatose and brain dead infants who are not autonomous. This is to say that Stenn's argument from the principle of autonomy is problematic and so it fails to give us a conclusive answer to the morality of euthanasia.

Likewise, Becker's argument from the principle of mercy cannot go unchallenged. Two major criticisms can be levelled against it. One can argue that due to scientific advancement in the field of medicine, there is now a "therapy" to pain. A patient can be given drugs which alleviate pain instead of practicing euthanasia on him her in the name of the principle of mercy-"the duty to act to end pain or suffering already occurring and the duty not to cause further pain or suffering"[2]. Thus, the principle of mercy can be said to be a thing of the past that in many cases can no longer be used as a justification to moralize euthanasia.

Besides, the principle of mercy is prone to abuse. As highlighted in the preceding discussion, some health professionals or home-care takers may feel burdened by a patient to the extent that they quicken the death of the patient in the name of the principle of mercy. This is to contend that the principle of mercy cannot absolutely justify the morality of euthanasia, hence its weakness.

Battin's argument that more forms of euthanasia should be allowed in America simply because the same has been done in other countries like Netherlands, can also be criticized. Actually, two criticisms can be levelled against her. The first one is that Battin's argument is fallacious. She commits *Argumentum ad populam*, a fallacy of appealing to the mob. This is because on logical grounds, a practice cannot be morally right for the one reason that it is being practiced in other cultures. Its moral status should depend on its validity and soundness, and not at all on individual tastes, inclinations or values upheld by a group of people. In this vein, Battin's argument cannot pass the logic of moral reasoning. As a matter of consequence, it cannot justify the morality of euthanasia.

From another angle, Battin's argument that more forms of euthanasia especially active euthanasia should be allowed on moral grounds can be rebutted. Have and Welie for instance, have argued that "euthanasia by the Dutch (in Netherlands) is largely unregulated. As a result, the number of cases of abuse is larger than people realize."[3] To stretch the argument further Have Welie contends that "physicians report that they engage in active euthanasia because they made a decision that the patient's case is hopeless rather than because they think that this is what the patient wants."[4] The two therefore conclude that allowing any form of active euthanasia opens the door for substantial abuse, especially when the physicians are faced with the task of continuing to treat a seriously ill patient. It (euthanasia) threatens the lives of patients even those whose diagnosis and prognosis of death can in due course, turn otherwise. It also results in lack of trust in health care professionals by patients and members of the public. Thus for these reasons, Battin's argument that active euthanasia should be allowed because it is practiced morally in other countries, can be laid to rest.

One final argument can be raised against those who argue for euthanasia. The argument has its roots in ancient Greece and the Hippocratic Oath which represents the tradition of oaths and codes, a version of which a physician took (and indeed takes) upon graduation form a Medical School, which condemned giving patients deadly drugs, "...neither will I administer a poison to anybody when asked to do so nor will I suggest such a case..."[5] This is to say that the message transmitted from one generation of doctors to the next (even to physicians of this day) was that physicians are supposed to be healers, not killers. To this end, euthanasia is considered morally wrong and everyone who practices it fails to fulfil the traditional goal of medicine.

A critique of arguments for euthanasia has been made. Let us now critically reflect on the arguments forwarded against euthanasia.

Critical Reflection on Con- euthanasia Arguments

Arguments against euthanasia, like those forwarded in favour of euthanasia, seem to have equally failed to convincingly respond to the question of the morality of euthanasia. The argument from the African perspective and that of Aquinas – argument from nature for instance, can be criticized for being rigid and narrow, that is, only based on culture and religion respectively. I shall treat these two arguments together because they are akin to each other. Though the arguments tally with the Biblical injunction "Do not kill,"[6] they seem to be narrow in their focus. They fail to realize that there are some cases which indeed warrant euthanasia even though euthanasia is not a fundamental right for anyone. For instances, cases of severely defective new-borns show that their (new-borns) prospective life is more than bad and no one seem to desire to live such kind of life. Suppose as sometimes happens:

46

A child is hydrocephalic with an extremely low intelligent quotient (IQ) is blind and deaf, has no control over its body, and can only lie on its back all day and have all its needs taken care of by others, and even cries out with pain when it is touched or lifted. Infants born with *spina bifida*- and this number over two per one thousand births- are normally not so badly off, but sometimes they are so.[7]

A crucial question arises here: "Would it be fair, just and humane to let live such an infant born with *spina bifida*, who would undoubtedly live a miserable and bad life?" I am of the view that it is unfair, unjust, inhumane and immoral to let such an infant live. One of course might ask. 'What criterion are we using in judging life as bad or good?'

To the projected question, Brandt seems to have a sound answer. He suggests that "one criterion to be used might be called a 'happiness' criterion for example if a person likes a moment of experience while he is having it his life is so far good, if a person dislikes a moment of experience while he is having it, his life is so far bad."[8] What Brandt is tantamount to saying is that based on such reactions, we might construct a "happiness curve" for a person. The curve would go up above the difference axis when a moment of experience is liked – and how far above depend on how strongly it is liked, and dipping down below the line when the moment is disliked. The criterion thus would say that a life is worth living if there is a net balance of positive area. All this is a clear testimony that the Africans and Aquinas' arguments are somehow narrow, rigid and consequently morally weak especially if we "are to think vividly of what kind of life the severely defective new-borns and also the comatose will have in any case."[9]

Like Aquinas' argument discussed above, Williams' first three arguments; argument from nature, argument from self-interest and argument from practical effects also seem to overlook the existence of some critical cases which would really warrant euthanasia. His last argument; the slippery slope argument cannot be as well excluded from this "mess". One might ask; "should individuals (such as the one born with *spina bifida* cited above) and the brain dead infants be made to suffer simply because if euthanasia is allowed in some cases, this will create a situation difficult to stop or control-a slippery slope situation?" A similar situation took place in Germany when the Nazi Germans terminated the lives of the Jews in the name of euthanasia. The situation was indeed very difficult to control until humanitarian groups intervened. Thus one may ask, "why (instead of allowing such a situation) not simply set stern and thought conditions in place which a case should satisfy for it to be considered as a case that warrant euthanasia?" I am convinced that though some would argue that the prospective lives of many defective new-borns are modestly pleasant such that it would be some injury to them to be terminated, justice will have been done if the lives of the severely defective new-borns are terminated. The major reason for holding this view is that the lives they will live are the ones many of us, if we are to be sure, would prefer not to live at all. To deny 'the right to die' to those defective new-borns with very critical circumstances would be therefore grossly unfair and morally unjust. I would rather suggest that very stern and well thought conditions should be set in place for those who would want their cases to count instead of taking William's extreme position which, in fact, appears to be rigid and dogmatic. I will stretch this argument a mile further in the next chapter.

The Problems and Dilemma of Euthanasia in Contemporary Africa: A Closer Look

Philosophers as far back as Plato have wrestled with complex or near impossible moral questions that test the character of the person making the decision. Today, these questions are known as moral dilemmas. It is curious, however to note that centuries of debate have left many of these dilemmas unsolved. In fact, moral dilemmas especially in practical philosophy like medical ethics have drastically increased over the past few decades.

The realization of the connection between the African traditional view of euthanasia and African traditional views is crucial. It helps us understand the African view of euthanasia, its strengths and weaknesses as a theory/view. It also helps us understand that in Africa, the stalemate brought forth by the clash between tradition and modern human right discussions have created new dilemmas- the 21st African euthanasia dilemma- an issue which in the past was never a dilemma. Thus today we now have the African dilemma on whether euthanasia should be allowed or not. While African traditional sanctification of life like other con-euthanasia arguments paraded in the previous discussion seems to offer a laudable justification for the continued existence of the status quo concerning euthanasia-disallowing euthanasia- inconsistencies and moral dilemmas surround the practice. Let us define a moral dilemma before looking at the African dilemma of euthanasia posed by the African traditional view of euthanasia.

A moral dilemma also known as an ethical dilemma is "a situation wherein moral precepts or ethical obligations conflict in such a way that any possible resolution to the dilemma is morally intolerable."[10] It is any situation in which a person making a decision experiences a conflict between moral oughts or guiding moral principles such that s/he cannot determine which course of action is right or wrong. Many times, moral dilemmas involve a morally wrong decision that produces a desirable result, or vice versa. Sometimes, they involve a decision in which the person is forced to choose only one of the two good things. One classic example of a moral dilemma is the famous 1842 shipwreck in which the captain was forced to choose between throwing the weak passengers overboard or letting all the passengers drown. Parading the dilemma in detail:

> In 1842, a ship is destroyed by an iceberg. Around 30 survivors are left and there is only a single lifeboat that has a capacity of 7 individuals. The weather is getting worse and the Captain of the ship has to decide how to lighten the boat so that at least the 7 people can survive. He is in a moral dilemma here. He decides that some of the individuals, mostly weaker people would have to be forced out of the boat. They will drown (which they eventually will) and the remaining 7 people will be safe at least[11].

Making an analysis of this situation, one would note that on one hand the captain's decision is totally reasonable as he wants to save the life of at least 7 people. But on the other hand he is killing 23 people to save these 7 which is immoral. Thus the decision is difficult and qualifies to pass as a moral dilemma. The 1982 movie *Sophie's Choice* portrays another moral dilemma, in which a mother is forced to choose which of her two children would be executed in a concentration camp.[12] Moral dilemmas take at least the following two general forms: 1). Some evidence indicates that act P is morally right, and some equally strong evidence indicates that act P is morally wrong. Abortion, for instance, is sometimes said to be a terrible modern moral dilemma for women who see the evidence this way and, 2). The agent believes that on moral grounds s/he both ought to and not ought to perform act P. In the contemporary age, euthanasia performed through intentional cessation of lifesaving therapies in the case of permanently comatose patients is considered dilemmatic in this second sense especially from an African point of view. This is what we shall call "the African dilemma of euthanasia", in this book. It should be noted that a conflict between a moral ought on one hand and self-interest on the other hand is not a moral dilemma but a practical dilemma. This is to say a moral dilemma only occurs when there are two moral ought/obligation that are in a sort of conflict in which an action that one ought to perform cannot be done without forgoing an equally important action.

The African dilemma of euthanasia has emerged as a result of the conceptions of euthanasia by critics of the African traditional of euthanasia on one hand, and the traditional custodians of African culture -conservatives- on the other hand. The complexities of these dilemmas are predicated on the difficulties faced by emerging African scholars in challenging traditional authority which is conceived as a holy grain, paragon of unquestionable authority. In spite of the disgruntlement and reservations about traditional practice of euthanasia, the practice continues unabated, notwithstanding its contradictions, in some cases, with individual rights of the defenceless patients. Yet some critical questions still remain unanswered: "Should we continue abiding by the African view of euthanasia or we should break away from the shackles of tradition? If we break away which position, then, should we adopt-allowing allowing all euthanasia cases or allow only some?" Whichever way, we remain with a moral dilemma. Continuing negating euthanasia may be considered as a failure to respect the moral integrity and values of individual patients. At the same time, allowing euthanasia as a trump to override the demands of the African traditional values and physicians values may require both traditionalists and physicians to act contrary to some of the most basic values of their culture and medicine respectively. The upshot is that the obligations generated by this situation result in moral dilemmas as it is extremely difficult as both perspectives seem to merit equal consideration.

At this juncture, some more critical questions arise: "Isn't it that if both perspectives (traditional values and individual rights) merit equal consideration, then, both are right? But can both perspectives be right? Isn't it ignorance that influences us to think that both perspectives require equal consideration?" I agree these questions like any philosophical question are not easy to tackle, but can be discussed. I would begin by reiterating that both pro- and con- euthanasia partisans seem to have failed to settle the question of euthanasia. On the other hand, the African view of euthanasia has been criticized for failing respect the moral integrity and values of individual patients. In fact, neither the western nor the African views of euthanasia have satisfactorily contributed as a strategy through which forces of medical ethics would benefit health professionals and the public in decision making on issues of euthanasia. Given such a scenario, an alternative theory is necessary. The virtue of the next chapter is therefore to ascertain how powerful and influential a moderate view of euthanasia as a vehicle for stimulating change and attitude in other researchers and public in general.

Notes

1. Mayor, F. *A history of Educational thought*, 3rd Ed, Merrill Publishing Company, Ohio, 1993, p.60.

2. Tom, l. Beauchamp. (ed), *Medical Ethics; The moral responsibilities of Physicians*, Prentice Hall, New Jersey, 1984, p. 14.

3. McDonald, M.J. *Contemporary Moral Issues in a Diverse Society*, Wadsworth Publishing Company, 1981, p. 159.

4. Larry May, (Ed), *Applied Ethics; A multicultural Approach*, Prentice Hall, New Jersey, 1994, p.489.

5. Jones, W.H.S. (Trans). *Hippocrates* "Selections from the Hippocratic Corpus" in Veatch, R. (Ed), *Cross Cultural Perspectives in Medical Ethics*, J & Burllett Publishers, Boston, 1989, p.29.

6. Exodus 20 v.13, *The Holly Bible, New International Version*, International Bible Society, Colorado, USA, 1984.

7. Brandt, R.B. 'Defective New-borns and the Morality of Termination' in Arthur, J. (Ed), *Morality and Moral Controversies*, 3rd Ed, Prentice Hall, New Jersey, 1993. p.160

8. Brandt, R.B. 1993. p.160.

9. Brandt, R.B. 1993. p.160.

10.
http://www.ehow.com/about.5481837/ethical.dilemma

11.   Tiffany   Bennett,   2010,
(http://www.ehow.com/about.5481837/ethical.dilemma

12.   Tiffany   Bennett,   2010,
(http://www.ehow.com/about.5481837/ethical.dilemma.

Chapter Four

Challenging the African Traditional View of Euthanasia: The 21st Century African Dilemma

The twenty first century African dilemma of euthanasia cannot be dismantled before looking at the basis of the African traditional view of euthanasia. And, maybe to understand better the African basis of euthanasia we need to understand the concept of tradition itself. The word tradition is derived from the Latin word *traditio* meaning to hand down or hand over. Tradition therefore means "customs, opinions, beliefs, legends, information, events, stories which have been passed to posterity –generation to generation-especially by word of mouth (orally) or by practice."[1] Tradition thus, generally means something that has been going on for a long time. Though the precision of the concept of tradition as opposed to modernity has come to be questioned by scholars like Bruno who argues that even Europeans have never been modern although they thought they were modern as they overstated their abilities to divorce themselves from their own traditions as there still exist some monarchies[2], the debate about modernity and tradition have been raging since the Enlightenment in Europe and subsequently in Africa. In Africa, as in Europe, the debate has been incited by disagreements between "conservative thinkers" and advocates of Enlightenment. The former pointing out the necessity of what were called traditional ways of life including the community and its values of communitarianism rather than individualism argued for the divine or nature to take its course in all spheres of life. On the other hand, advocates of the Enlightenment made a case for what has come to be called progress, associated with modernity, rationality, logic, empiricism, human rights, equality, freedom including freedom from the tyranny of monarchical authority and traditional beliefs. Thus, tradition was associated with conservatism – with the unwillingness to change, stagnation, superstition, irrationality and authoritarianism – while modernity was associated with change, secularization, freedom/liberty, rationality and progress.

Drawing on the understanding of tradition above, it can be remarked that there are various different traditions around and some could be considered as slightly strange, whilst others are used by thousands of different people. Overall a tradition is something that means a lot to those that abide by it such that breaking or violating it may result in sanctions or serious consequences from the group, society or custodians of the tradition. It is this element of tradition that makes it difficult for most Africans to think otherwise when it comes to the question of euthanasia.

In African societies in general, it is a truism that treatment of individual lives as sacred and the relegation of euthanasia can foster a cohesive and united society if pragmatically applied. That is, when founded on the foundations informed by respect of goodwill, principle of autonomy, custodianship, individual rights, societal solidarity and mutual dependence, rather than obsession with tradition, abuse of privilege and suppression of individual and civil rights. Due to the oppressive nature of the African view of euthanasia and misinterpretation of euthanasia by African traditionalists in contemporary Africa, critics assert that it constitutes a crime against humanity as it perpetuates human suffering, individual human right violations and deeply asymmetrical relations of power in what is supposedly an egalitarian society.

It is in this light that I challenge the African traditional view of euthanasia that seems deeply anchored in misinterpretation of the moral nature and integrity of mankind. African traditionalists misconstrue communalism as the same authority that is bestowed to them by virtue of the position they occupy as cultural administrators that connects the living and the living dead/ the spiritual realm. They have manipulated this opportunity to impose disguised "paternalism" that is firmly rooted in unparalleled hegemony and self-enrichment to the extent that Africans who hold different views on euthanasia have remained fearful to challenge the status quo. Yet, the African traditional view of euthanasia is founded merely on African communalism which prioritizes community values over individual values and integrity. Critical questions therefore remain: "Isn't that by letting community values overriding those of the individuals, we are merely advancing the values of the custodians of culture at the expense of those of some community members? Isn't it more appropriate to consider integrity and values of each community member first before those of the community?"

Thus, in contemporary times punctuated by numerous terminal diseases, accidents of all forms, infants born with *spina bifida* in Africa and the world over, the patients and indeed the public are caught in the horns of a dilemma. The dilemma is whether they could object to a practice traced from historical tradition as a source of venerating life and upholding communal values on the one hand, and insulating themselves from oppressive nature of the traditional/cultural view of euthanasia, on the other. As rightly noted by Roger E.

57

Barker, "a child is born culture-free; one is born into a culture."[3] Yet while it is truism that one may assume the culture into which s/he is born, it is equally important to emphasize that breaking away from tradition is momentous for any normal human being. However, this cannot serve as a foundation for unjust human suffering especially even where alternatives are conceivably limited.

I infer from this understanding that in such tension between preservation of tradition riddled with manipulations and continuity with global values of mankind that threatens lives of the patients, panaceas are hard to come by. In this light, it is imperative that the Governments of African countries and independent organizations intervene so that the traditional view of euthanasia is absolved, reconstituted or reconstructed or rather re-worked on foundations informed by respect of goodwill, principle of autonomy, individual rights, societal solidarity and mutual dependence. A moderate view of euthanasia is one example of such a view that is informed by respect of goodwill, principle of autonomy, individual rights, societal solidarity, mutual dependence and above all reason.

Towards a Moderate View of Euthanasia

From the previous discussion, it is apparent that in this twenty first century where human rights discussions have taken a new direction, there is great need to advance fresh views to tackle head the contentious issue of euthanasia. A moderate view of euthanasia is therefore proposed in place of the two extreme, seemingly rigid and opposed views of euthanasia explicated previously in this book. In general terms, the moderate view of euthanasia acknowledges that euthanasia is not a fundamental "right" for anyone but at the same time each case should be considered special in its own right. That said, each case should be treated differently depending on circumstances surrounding it. The moral rightness or wrongness of euthanasia or the "ought" is therefore determined by the circumstances that surround the case in question. This view has the advantage that it promotes what we call "negotiated justice", where a just decision is rationally made not only by one person/part but through negotiation by many parties. More so, it [moderate view of euthanasia] gives advantage to all kind of patients, the competent and incompetent ones; hence its merit over both the pro-and con-euthanasia arguments.

To concretize the aforementioned view of euthanasia, this work makes reference to four "exemplary cases" which indeed warrant a moderate view of euthanasia as both pro- and con-euthanasia views cannot separately give a "fair" and sound response to the referred. The first one has been highlighted in the preceding paragraphs; the case of severely defective new-borns. I have already argued that severely defective new-borns undoubtedly live bad life and so it would be a favour to them if their lives were terminated. Of course one might argue that "it is not for their (severely defective infants) sake but to avoid trouble to others that they are allowed to die."[4] But I remained convinced that such patients as brain dead infants and those infants born with *spina bifida*, among others, live bad life- the kind of life which if we think vividly of what it will be like in any case, none of us would prefer it. But still, two mind boggling questions can be raised; 'if a decision to terminate a severely new-born is to be morally acceptable, how soon must it be made and the conclusion be effected? And, which defects should be considered severe and serious that they would definitely call for euthanasia?'

In response to the first question, Brandt suggested "the time of termination should not be postponed to the age of five or of three or even a year."[5] This is because at these ages all the reasons for insisting on consent are already cogent. It can therefore be recommended that if life is to be terminated, this should be done within ten days especially given that doubtless advances in medicine will permit detection of serious prospective defects early in pregnancy.

In view of the second question, it seems obvious that guidelines after thorough analysis of the case under consideration must be established. Lorber proposed five guidelines he said should be used as a yardstick to judge the prospective life of a defective infant. Firstly, he considers the cases of *spina bifida*. He notes that "if this is on the lower half of the back, the baby will be severely paralyzed and incontinent and probably have severe hydrocephalus."[6] The second condition considered by Lorber is paralysis whereby if a baby is paralyzed at birth, it will never recover its muscle power. The third is gross distortion of the spine as a result of, for example, *kyphosis*. He notes that "those new-borns affected by paralysis are among the most handicapped children and the consequences tend to worsen with time."[7] Fourthly, Lorber does consider the condition of gross hydrocephalus. The fifth and last condition Lorber considers concerns other gross congenital malformations along with *bina fida*. After outlining these guidelines, Lorber argues that a child with any of these conditions should not be recommended for treatment but should be let dying. It should be emphasized that Lorber is not advocating for the termination of all defective infants but only those infants with

60

conditions stated above. This is to contend that even though Lorber did not go further to explicitly pronounce and advance the view advanced by this work (a moderate view) , a moderate view of euthanasia seem necessary and worth adopting in dealing with some critical cases.

Let us consider yet another case: A soldier in the past US and UK war against Iraq has been fatally injured. He has bullets in the skull, both legs and hands amputated, eyes plucked off, and have sustained other injuries all over the body which are continually bleeding and hardly dry-up. He is also experiencing persisting unbearable pain which causes him to spend sleepless nights. And worse still, he has lost his sanity that he is no longer competent. Now considering the life of this soldier, taking note that his life is seemingly miserable, bad and hopeless; would it, then, be morally right to allow him to live? Surely, this is a somehow trick and no easy question. One may argue that the life that one considers to be miserable, bad and hopeless might be considered vice versa by the patient concerned. The researcher however thinks that this could not be so with the patient presented in the case above even if he is financially sound to survive by the respiratory system. To substantiate this view, it can be argued that any normal rational being with a fair mind can easily judge that the patient (soldier) is undoubtedly living a "miserable life"- a life that the patient himself truly feels is bad and hopeless. The patient can no longer bath, walk, or even feed by himself. He can no longer enjoy discussions with his fellow comrades. What happy moment can he therefore enjoy in his life?

In a case as this, if one is to employ Brandt's criterion (explicated in the preceding paragraphs) of judging life as bad or good – the "happiness criterion", it will be revealed that the enjoyments, if ever there, being experienced by the patient are brief if ever any. They can hardly balance the long stretches of boredom, discomfort and pain the patient is experiencing. For this reason, one can speculate that on the whole, the patient's life is undoubtedly miserable; one that many of us would prefer not to live at all. The researcher therefore is of the view that even though the victim cannot consent, his fellow comrades can still make a decision on his behalf which they think is altruistic and would be in accordance with his best wishes had it been that he was competent. In this case, though euthanasia is not a right for anyone, a decision can be made that the patient's life be terminated for his own sake (considering his situation). This conclusion clearly shows that a moderate view of euthanasia should be adopted; each case should be treated differently.

Another case (this is a real not a hypothetical case) is that of a 120 year old man. The old man, due to old age no longer sees walks, eats, baths and sit on his own. He is always asleep. No one knows when he is happy, sad, ill or what a view, for he no longer hears or recognizes the voices of the people, even those whom he lives with. He has also lost his competence. The man, in fact, is no longer able to do anything on his own. He cannot even know whether it is night or day time. A critical question can be raised: "Which is morally better to let the man 'rest' or to keep him living?"

The case just referred to is indeed tricky and no easy to solve. However, like the soldier's case, the old man seems to be living an uncomfortable life (even if we are to use Brandt's happiness criterion) that many of us would not prefer to live at all. I therefore think that though the victim can no longer consent, his fellow comrades and "other parties" can still make a decision on his behalf (to apply passive euthanasia on him) which they think is altruistic and would be in accordance with his best wishes had it been that he was competent. This is not to say that euthanasia should be applied to all old people.

One final case may still be introduced; A 70 year old woman is in hospital seriously suffering from incurable diseases, HIV/AIDS, epilepsy and asthma. She is experiencing terrible perennial pain which makes her spend sleepless nights. She now has wounds all over and is getting thin every day. Worst of all, her condition no longer allows her to walk, bath and feed alone. Now, knowing for certain that she is going to die in the near future yet she is spending the little resources (on medication) which her children could use later, and that she is burdening those who are nursing her, the woman requests to have the respirator disconnected and her life be terminated. She has been judged competent. A question now can be raised; "should the patient be allowed to have her life terminated?" Here the duty to preserve life is in direct conflict with the principle of mercy and the duty to respect one's autonomy. All are prima facie duties and to fix the actual duty becomes extremely difficult. It will however be suggested that the patient's choice should be allowed to override the duty to preserve life because considerations of autonomy are here, though not everywhere, weightier. More so, it can still be argued that most if not all people would like to die a dignified death. Yet studies on HIV/AIDS patients have shown that majority of AIDS patients die in abject poverty, unable to buy the food and medication they need.[8] This is because HIV/AIDS patients normally require very expensive package of treatment that the already financially burdened family members can no longer manage, given the long illness and the financial costs that goes with it. The state of hopelessness brought forth by HIV/AIDS strips them of human dignity and is not worth it.

Besides, HIV/AIDS patients and their caregivers or family members face public humiliation, social rejection and stigmatization in many African societies. Stigmatization is a complex social and psychological process whereby certain persons are perceived as without social value, even threatening the well-being of the dominant society.[9] This is because outsiders identify the HIV/AIDS patients with their family members. As such, they have a tendency of treating both the infected and the family members with fear of being infected through association. In most African societies, for example in Mozambique, Zimbabwe, Swaziland, Malawi and Zambia among other African countries, if a member of a given family is known to be an HIV/AIDS patient, the whole family, especially the caregivers, the spouse and children, are shunned by many because of the fear of getting infected. The same fear also makes physicians, though may accept treating HIV/AIDS patients, reluctant to treat them with a high degree of "seriousity". This makes HIV/AIDS patients and their family members feel socially rejected and discriminated against by other members of their society. Despite campaigns to demystify the beliefs held by most people on how HIV/AIDS is transmitted, it remains difficult for most Africans to associate or even shake hands with an HIV/AIDS patient for fear of being infected. This even aggravates the patient's situation by making his/her life even more difficult as the patient will have to endure the incurable disease, social rejection and stigmatization. Given that both home-based care initiatives and medicine itself have failed to totally solve the multiplicity of challenges being faced by HIV/AIDS patients in Africa and beyond, it can be argued that when one's quality of life goes down as a result of chronic and terminal illness and suffering, the moderate view of euthanasia is necessary to evaluate if the desire to continue living can be overridden by a desire to quit life. For these reasons, I believe the effectiveness of the African view of euthanasia and con-euthanasia position in the context of a disease that has no known cure to date, is questionable. I therefore suggest that a moderate view of view of euthanasia is worth considering in some cases of euthanasia. In the case under consideration, it would seem morally right to allow the patient, for her own sake to "have a rest" as per her wish. This would enable her to escape from the life-long misery of pain and thinking about her own health status and family.

In a nutshell, I am strongly convinced that in cases such as those presented above [cases 1-4], a moderate view of euthanasia is necessary, deserving to be seriously considered by the medical fraternity and by members of the public. It helps us to deal with the critical situations of "some" patients easier as compared to the two opposing views (pro-and con-euthanasia arguments) paraded in the prior discussions which seem to be rigid, dogmatic and narrowly focused. However, one should note that this is not to argue that euthanasia should be applied to all cases of patients lest it will be as good as arguing that euthanasia is a fundamental right for everyone or is morally right in all circumstances. Instead, this work advances the argument that each case should be treated differently depending on its unique circumstances not just giving the same respond to all cases- giving a "no" or a "yes" to all euthanasia cases. For example, in cases where pain is short-lived, where there is a possibility of an inaccurate prognosis of death, where a patient is suffering from a curable or where a patient's condition is not severe (even is suffering from an incurable disease), where there are possibilities that a patient can recover and other such cases; a moderate view euthanasia should not apply even if the person asking for euthanasia is judged competent. But in special cases as those cited above patients should be accorded the right to "choose death". This is to say in special cases as 1, 2, 3, and 4, the "right to choose death" like the "right to life" should be recognized as one of the human rights and civil rights to be accorded members of society. This is what Donnelly suggests when he remarks: "human rights are those basic standards without which people cannot live in dignity;"[10] the rights or entitlements one has, for the plain reason that s/he is a human being. It is from this understanding that one can infer that patients in situations cited above are no longer living in dignity meaning they are being deprived of some human rights.

The Principle of Beneficence

Besides the cases I have presented to justify a moderate view of euthanasia, the prima facie principle of beneficence can be forged to defend a moderate view of euthanasia. This is because beneficence often creates an obligation for physicians to consider the patient's best interests rather than those of the physician where the law is silent. The word beneficence broadly used in English mean the doing of good, the active promotion of good, kindness and charity. More commonly in medical ethics, beneficence is understood as "a principle requiring that physicians provide positive benefits such as health as well as prevent and remove harmful conditions from patients."[11] In other words, the principle asserts an obligation to help others further their important

66

and legitimate interests, and abstain from injuring them. It should be remarked that the obligation to confer benefits and actively prevent and remove harms is important in biomedical ethics, but equally important is the obligation to weigh and balance the possible goods against the possible harms of an action.[12] This makes it appropriate to distinguish two principles under the general principle of beneficence. The first is called the principle of positive beneficence since it requires the provision of benefits including the prevention and removal of harm as well as promotion of welfare. The second is a version of the principle of utility. It requires a balancing of benefits and harms in moral life.[13] Considering the latter principle of beneficence-principle of utility- the ancient source of the principle of beneficence appears in a central passage from the Hippocratic Oath which says: "I will apply dietetic measures to the benefit of the sick according to my ability and judgment; I will keep them from harm and injustice."[14] This statement acknowledges the physician's special knowledge and skills as well as his/her commitment to principles requiring the use of those skills in order to benefit patients. But what benefit can a physician guarantee a patient in case 1 to 4 above who are terminally ill and living a life that any person with an average mind would describe as miserable? Isn't it that assisting them escaping their incessant sufferings would be the greatest benefit a physician can render a patient besides his/her knowledge to cure curable diseases of patients? It is my conviction that in such situations as those paraded in cases 1-4 above assisting the patient to rest for good would benefit the patient more than letting him/her continue living in anguish. This line of reasoning enjoys support from other portions of the Hippocratic writings which give a fuller account of the

67

perspective from which acting in the patient's best interest is to be understood. In the passage from *The Art*, the Hippocrates has this to say, "I will define what I conceive medicine to be. In general terms, it is to do away with the suffering of the sick, to lessen the violence of their diseases, and to refuse to treat those who are overmastered by their diseases, realizing that in such cases medicine is powerless."[15] I infer from this passage that where medicine can no longer be of any benefit to the patient as in the case of patients 1, 2, 3 and 4 cited above. It will be to the benefit of the patient to assist him/her to rest for good, hence the justification of the moderate view of euthanasia.

While the principle of beneficence has gone a mile to justify the plausibility of a moderate view of euthanasia, we can still employ the principle of "negotiated justice" to ground its logicality. But before considering the latter principle we will examine Rawls' theory of justice from which the principle was adopted.

Rawls' Theory of Justice

The concept of justice, though a critical one and its importance was far more recognized by social and political philosophers of the past perhaps than it is by those of the present, it remains a confusing and troublesome concept for social and political philosophy and philosophy in general. As such, the concept of justice has received different interpretations throughout history from as far back as the time of Plato. For purposes of this work, we will however, not delve into details of the discussions of definitions given by different scholars over the years. We will only look, of course briefly, at the concept of justice this book identifies with. The book identifies with John Rawls' theory of justice. I should not be mistaken to claim that Rawls' theory of justice is the best or the only theory of justice that can be explored with regards to euthanasia and medical ethics in general. It is of course as good a starting point as any other theory of justice. However, one of the virtues of Rawls' theory of justice is that it is rich in content and, accordingly, can be applied successfully to various medical ethics related issues.

In his *A Theory of Justice*, first published in 1971, John Rawls formulated one of the most influential theories of justice and social and political ethics published in the last three and half decades. Though the theory was intended to protect the rights of individual persons from "political bargaining" or "the calculus of social,"[16] his theory is partly a response to the consequentialist theory-utilitarianism-which call for the greatest happiness for the greatest number, but does not exclude the possibility of leaving out a minority unhappy. Instead, Rawls understands justice as "fairness"[17] where at the initial stage/situation all men have equal liberty, social status and opportunity to natural asserts/chief primary goods. This does not mean to say the concepts of justice and fairness are the same. Instead, this means that justice as fairness "begins with one of the most general of all choices which persons will make together with the choice of the first principles of a conception of justice which is to regulate all subsequent criticism and reform of situations"[18]. Thus Rawls' just society is based on rational and disinterested principles contracted by all society and with mutual consent of the latter [all society] in a hypothetical original position of equality and freedom, a position Rawls himself calls "the veil of ignorance"[19]. The veil of ignorance is an imaginary device that can be used to determine what is fair in society, that is, to determine everyone's advantage and liberty. Rawls came to this conclusion after realizing that it is part of human nature; 1) "to be rational- to take the most effective means to given ends and, 2) to look out for personal interest –not taking an interest in one another's interests in the sense of allowing others the liberty and opportunity to fulfil different plans than one's own."[20] A strong point Rawls is making here is that "if people acting from self-interest are able to choose principles of justice emphasizing fairness, i.e. equal liberty and opportunity, it seems anyone else would."[21] For Rawls, behind the veil of ignorance, everyone has the general knowledge for determining what principles of justice will regulate society in future, but lacks knowledge about his/her own individual case. In other words, no one in the imagined state of Rawls is in possession of prejudicial information, that is, knowledge which would allow him/her to hold for principles which would benefit him/her if s/he knew what his/her position was to be [in the present and in the future]. Basing on this, Rawls assumes, the only rational choice that self-interested people behind the veil of ignorance can make about the principles of justice in society is giving equal liberty and equal opportunity to all. This will be the only way to guarantee that everyone will receive a relatively good life as this kind of justice ensures that no one is advantaged or disadvantaged as all are similarly situated such that no one is able to design principles to his/her favour. Justice in this sense is conceived as the opposite of injustice which is simply "inequalities that are not to the benefit of all."[22] In this latter situation the principles of justice are not agreed to in an initial situation that is fair or in a situation that is reached by a fair agreement or bargain between individuals.

The Principle of Negotiated Justice

From Rawls' theory of justice as fairness, this work adopts some of the assumptions and considerations in order to develop a principle of medical ethics we shall call "negotiated justice". This principle can be applied by the moderate view to help decide and settle troublesome euthanasia questions I am certain are deeply rooted in the life experiences of most of the people of Africa and those beyond the borders of the continent. These questions are:

1). How do we resolve the problem where personal autonomy clash with communal values.

2). If a moderate view of euthanasia is adopted, who should judge euthanasia cases?

3). Under what circumstances can a case pass as a euthanasia case and vice versa?

These questions are not only critical to those concerned with the issue of euthanasia, but they are troublesome for medical ethics. With this principle a "fair judgment" on the patient's case is reached through negotiations by various parties not only the patient or the physician or the patient's family alone. By "negotiated justice", I mean therefore a fair decision reached by various parties through negotiations and democratic processes or free will. It is justice executed by many and through democratic means. The latter may involve balloting/voting besides open discussions motivated by free will and not compulsion. Taking into account this understanding of justice, I suggest that the deliberation of a euthanasia case should be made through serious negotiations and a democratic process by a euthanasia council which comprises various parties, that is, people from different social orientations. These may include the patient (in the case of a competent patient), the patient's family, moral philosophers, physicians, independent/non-governmental organizations, government officials, religious leaders, village elders/chiefs, human rights organizations among others. If the council deems just and judges that it is in the interest of the patient to have euthanasia administered on him/her, then, the case should pass. And the council judges no, then the case should not pass. This is to say that euthanasia should not be considered neither as a fundamental right for humanity nor otherwise. Each case should be considered special in its own right. As such, what count when judging whether a case should pass or not are the circumstances surrounding each case.

Notes

1. Tradition, (http://www.blurtit.com).

2. Bruno Latour. 2007, 'The Recall of Modernity', *Cultural Studies Review*, 13, No. 1.

3. Roger E. Barker. *Education_and related concepts*, College Press Publishers, Harare, 1994, p.50.

4. Brandt, R.B. "Defective New-borns and the Morality of Termination" in Arthur, J. (Ed), *Morality and Moral Controversies*, Prentice Hall, 1993. p.164.

5. Brandt, R.B, 1993. p.165.

6. Brandt, R.B, in Arthur, J. (Ed), 1993, p.165.

7. Brandt, R.B, in Arthur, J. (Ed), 1993, p.165.

8. Katabira, E., Mubiru, F., & van Praag, E. Care for People Living with HIV/AIDS. In: Global Health Challenge:

Essays on AIDS. Commonwealth Secretariat: London, 2001, p.2.

9. Jonsen, A.R. "The Duty to Treat Patients with AIDS and HIV Infection" in Arras, J. D. and Steinbock, B. (Eds). *Ethical Issues in Modern Medicine*. Mayfield Publishing Company: London, 1995, p. 97-114.

10. Donnelley, J., Universal Human Rights in Theory and Practice, Cornell University Press, USA, 2003.

11. Tom L. Beauchamp. (Ed), *Medical Ethics: The Moral Responsibilities of Physicians*, Prentice Hall, New Jersey, 1984, p27.

12. Tom L. Beauchamp and Childress J.F., Principles of Biomedical Ethics, 3rd Ed, Oxford University Press, 1989, p.195.

13. Tom L. Beauchamp and Childress J.F, 1989, p.195.

14. Tom L. Beauchamp. (Ed). *Medical Ethics; The Moral Responsibilities of Physicians*, Prentice Hall, New Jersey, 1984, p.29.

15. Jones, W.H.S. (Trans), *Hippocrates* "Selections from the Hippocratic Corpus-The Art" vol. 11, in Veatch, R. (Ed), *Cross Cultural Perspectives in Medical Ethics*, J & Burllett Publishers, Boston, 1989, p.193.

16. See Manning R. 1981, Environmental Ethics and John Rawls' Theory of Justice, Journal of Environmental Ethics, vol. 3, 1981, p.155-165.

17. John Rawls, "A Theory of Justice", in Daniel Kolak, *Questioning Matters*, Mayfield Publishing Company, 1999, p.628.

18. John Rawls, 1999, p. 629.

19. John Rawls, 1999, p. 629.

20. John Rawls, 1999, p. 629.

21. See Pritchard M.S. and Robison W. L. 'Justice and the Treatment of Animals: A Critique of Rawls, Environmental Ethics', vol. 3, 1981, p. 61.

22. John Rawls, 1999, p. 631.

Chapter Five

Medical Doctors' Strike

Though physicians strike provides an opportunity to generate more knowledge about the process in which legitimacy of an organization can be restored, it meets with a great deal of resistance not only by the public but from within the medical profession. This chapter critically examines the legitimacy of strike by medical doctors heretofore referred to as physicians. While critically reflecting on strikes of physicians in general, this work makes more emphasis on Africa where physician strikes are rampant. More importantly, the work argues that strike implies a failure for everyone in the organization (including the strikers themselves), not only the responsible government or authority. This is because when a strike occurs, an organization/fraternity is subjected to questions, scrutiny and slander. It becomes difficult to decouple what is said, decided and done. Traditionally, all medical fraternities the world-over are committed to acting comfortably to external demands- guaranteeing the patients' lives and public health. By paying attention to external reactions, the medical fraternity adapts and learns what ought and should be done so that it is never again caught in the same messy. At the same time, the fraternity prepares itself for the future strikes. When the fraternity and those outside consider it is doing up to the external expectations, its lost legitimacy is restored. When legitimacy is restored, external pressure like once disturbed water returns to normal.

Background to Strikes in the Medical Fraternity

While there is monumental literature on pro-strike arguments on the one hand and con- strike arguments on the other, there is patchy literature that examines the nexus between the preservation of medical professionalism through African traditional beliefs/practices and the safeguard of human rights of the ordinary patients against physician strike actions. At best, academics have conceived these constituencies of academic research as irreconcilable research spheres that are beyond compromise. Drawing on the conception of physician strikes in Africa and the world-over, this work contributes to this grey area by demonstrating that the prestrike arguments have been extreme, narrowly focused and riddled with injustices. On the other hand, the anti-strike arguments based on the Hippocratic Oath need reconstruction or reconstitution or both; otherwise they cannot be accepted as well on philosophical grounds. It is worth noting at this juncture that all physician strike actions take place within an institution/medical fraternity which has a structure, a set of policies, a culture/tradition and a set of factual decision-making. Yet, the fraternity's tradition and set of policies among other things are violated when a strike occurs. When this happens some blame the physicians and others praise them; hence making strike actions a contested terrain. It is this light that the issue deserves incisive intellectual investigation, especially in an African context where incidences of strikes are rampant. The intractable nature of physician strike action heretofore referred to as strike makes it at root ethical and, in part, economic. It is in part economic because it deals with a group of professionals who offer their services for a price. And it is at root ethical in so far as it concerns itself with human behaviour and conduct and the difference between right and wrong, good and bad. This denotes that strike does not deal solely with factual judgments which can be said to be either true or false; hence its complexity. Consequently, the question on strike has become a common game for almost everybody- moralists, economists, academicians, national governments and the public. It has also become one of the most contentious of contemporary issues in the medical fraternity. This chapter conceptually analyses strike before advancing a con-strike argument based on four views/theories namely: utilitarianism, modified Hippocratic Oath and African communalism and the principle of beneficence. The sacrosanct of human life as is negatively undermined and threatened by physicians strike necessitated the research of this nature. Using the aforesaid theories, the book makes an attempt to demonstrate through "cases" drawn mainly from Africa the plausibility of con-strike view. This view is useful in that it pays veneration to the sanctity of life and promotes the majority's happiness. It also represents a human right oriented response from a patient and the public's perspective. More importantly, the emancipator approach of this book uses 'exemplary cases' to demonstrate how we can seek to understand the impact of strikes from credence values of beneficence, mercy and simple logic. This work therefore is an attempt to integrate African communalism, utilitarianism and the principle of civil rights and a modified version of the Hippocratic Oath into the main stream of physicians' strike discourse. In most if not all countries, this is necessary because in the name of physicians' strike, unnecessary deaths and sufferings of the public are inevitable. And civil rights are often violated and neglected, yet there are long term advantages to be gained by actively promoting them. In short, the virtue of this chapter is to ascertain how useful and influential the anti-strike view based on African communalism, the principle of beneficence, utilitarianism and modified Hippocratic Oath is, especially as a strategy where forces of medical ethics would essentially benefit healthy professionals, the public and their national governments in decision making relevant to the medical fraternity. The work thus, is a contribution towards efforts by those who are against physicians strike. It shifts emphasis from the dominant Western view on physician strike based on the old version of the Hippocratic Oath to the view against physicians strike as understood from the standpoints of African communalism, the principle of beneficence, utilitarianism and a modified Hippocratic Oath. It should be quickly noted, however, that the answer to the moral problems surrounding physician strike is very difficult to stipulate; thus the role of judging and deciding problems facing physicians should not be solely accredited to physicians alone, nor should it be accredited to the government alone. Instead, many parties such as non-governmental organizations, moralists, members of the public, patient committee, physicians and academics and the national government should contribute before a final deliberation to go on strike is made. The intricacies surrounding the question of physicians strike can best be disentangled and cogently dealt with only after attention is paid to the concept "strike" itself. This concept thus shall be discussed briefly before looking at the question on the morality and legitimacy of physicians strike; otherwise, the entire task of this work would tantamount to chasing the wind.

Conceptual analysis of strike

Strike is an issue in the medical fraternity that has aroused the interest of many professional ethicists, academicians and the public in general. Though often used as a bargaining tactic for most of the workers in the world-over, the concept is deeply controversial, for moral and practical reasons especially when dealt with in relation with physicians or workers in the medical fraternity in general. A number of interpretations to the term have been provided by scholars. Some have generally considered striking as a bargaining tactic by workers. Others have understood it as "self-contradictory action by". However, besides these generalizations, various attempts to formulate a workable definition of this obscure term have been made. Marxist-Leninist regimes such as the former USSR or the People's Republic of China define strike as a counter-revolutionary action-an action by workers against themselves.[1] Contrary to this sense, http://www.direct.gov.uk/en/Employment/TradeUnion/in dex.htm, defines strike action as a work stoppage caused by the mass refusal of employees to work. Strike can also be defined as "industrial dispute."[2] The differences between the definitions above suggest the reason why there is no consensus on the morality and legitimacy of strikes. It can however be argued that these definitions are ambiguous, because they do not make any reference to reasons that give rise to a strike. Also, the definitions does not make reference to who the strike is executed against, hence the need for a more encompassing and comprehensive definition. In this view, I shall define strike as mass refusal of employees to work according to their employment contract in response to an injustice(s) against them by their employer or in response to their grievances with the employer. It is curious to note that strike is one of the two forms (besides action short of strike such as 'go-slows', 'call-outs' or overtime bans) of industrial action; hence the need to define the latter. Industrial action is an action whereby members of a trade union are involved in a dispute with their employer that cannot be resolved by negotiation.[3]

Clashing views on physicians' strike

The question on whether physicians should go on strike or not has so far received different interpretations. It is indeed a contested terrain. Different interpretations have been conjured, yet no consensus has been reached. Two main camps have however been prominent since the late 19th and early 20th centuries when most western countries partially legalized striking.[4] While some people are against the idea of physicians going on strike, others support the idea as long as physicians feel they are being unjustly treated by their employer. In the face of such varied modes, it is perhaps unwise to attempt to reflect on the question on physicians' strike before paying some attention to the views given so far against and in favour of physicians' strike from whence the aforesaid camps ensue. Yet, it is a truism that only one and not both views for and against physicians' strike can be right. In is therefore the contention of this work that some of the previous researches on the issue under consideration were erroneous and others inadequate; hence the need to re-examine their assumptions and contributions. In the ensuing paragraphs, two camps on physicians' strikes, pro- strike and con-strike arguments, thus, shall be discussed briefly and separately in an attempt to determine the most plausible and philosophically convincing position.

The Pro- Physicians Strike View(s)

Negative scholarship on the idea of physicians going on strike has recently emerged. Robert Nozick and Beauchamp, for example, have initiated what unfortunately will be a growing trend of promoting the idea that physicians should go on strike whenever they deem necessary. What is distinctive of these scholars is that their approach is enormously economic. They seem to have been driven by a somewhat biased capitalistic philosophy which undermines morality, religion and all perspectives linked to Afro-centric philosophy. Such philosophers cannot be expected to be genuinely seeking the truth about the ethic-economical issue of physicians' strike. Beauchamp, for example, argues that physicians should go on strike whenever they deem necessary. In his words:

> Any system that favours the idea that physicians have ethical obligations that transcend self-interest, exigency and even political and economic forces is evaluated as capricious and unjust in so far as it fails to determine how social burdens and benefit sought to be allocated."[5]

It is interesting to note that, for Beauchamp, if the government or any system responsible for physicians' salaries fails to cohere with conventional standards and, to recognize their valuable social contribution, need and ambition, the latter are morally justified to go on strike. For him, strike is a way of reacting against an injustice of social, political, religious or economic nature. To this effect, his argument appeals to the principle of justice; hence the need to understand justice. For purposes of this study, the researcher shall identify with Pellegrino and Thomasma who define justice as the habit of rendering what is due to others[6]. For example, if a patient in a hospital deserves treatment to be cured of his/her disease, justice is done if and only if the patient receives the right treatment at the right time. The example given above shows that one who has a claim based on justice has a claim of entitlement. In this strong sense, the patient given in the example is due to something. An injustice, in turn, is done if s/he is denied to that s/he is entitled, in this case, treatment. It is in this light that physicians all over the world feel morally justified going on strike whenever they feel they are unjustly being treated by the government or authority responsible for their grievances. Although physicians are few of the most highly paid professionals in Africa and the world-over, those in developing countries still feel short-changed and unjustly paid; hence involved in strikes most of the time. Yet, questions that worry the critics and even the friends of strike partisans can be posed: What is so special about physicians as professionals that besides being the most highly paid professionals in most countries they still think they are unjustly paid? And is it morally justifiable to pay them "hefty salaries" when the majority of the people (as in the case of most developing countries) are suffering from abject poverty? To answer the question, we must know what justice is and, by what method/criteria we should judge an action as just. In view of the above raised question, John Rawls who understands justice as "fairness"[7] argues that: "What persons are entitled to or can legitimately claim is based on certain morally relevant properties they possess, such as being productive or being in great need (scarce). It is wrong, as a matter of justice, to burden someone if the person possesses the relevant property."[8]

Transposing this argument to the issue of physicians, it can be argued that physicians possess morally relevant properties insofar as they are a scarce resource, productive and greatly needed. It is out of this understanding that Beauchamp and Rawls argue that physicians are morally justified to go on strike if they are not happy with their wages or conditions of service. A lingering question(s) arises at this juncture: Does the fact physicians have morally relevant properties makes their strike a morally justifiable act? And does the morally relevant properties of physicians justify them gaining economic advantage over other professionals abiding by similar existing societal principles and values?' Nozick reasons along with Beauchamp and Rawls in support of physician's strike. He employs a libertarian theory of justice. In his words a government's action is justified if and only if it protects the rights the rights or entitlements of citizens, the right of citizens not to be coerced.[9] But in the medical fraternity whose rights to respect? Should it be those of physicians or those of patients or both? In view of this question, Nozick is tempted to reason that the rights of both should be preserved; however, those of doctors should be preserved first if justice is to prevail. For him, satisfying the needs and interests of physicians would in turn satisfy those of patients. His argument can be understood through the following logic: 1) If the needs and interests of physicians are satisfied, physicians will in turn satisfy the interests and needs of the patients; 2) Physicians' needs and interests are satisfied. Therefore the patients' needs and interests are satisfied. It is curious however, to note that Nozick's argument is a contemporary malaise -one based on haste generalization for it is possible that physicians' needs and interests are satisfied yet the latter still fails to satisfy the patients' needs and interests. It is therefore surprising and disturbing that Nozick strongly believes that if government satisfies the needs and interests of physicians, it is acting justly to all citizens, even the patients and the public in general. In this light, the paper contends that physicians strike is never morally good and justifiable on the basis of Nozick's argument. A critical question can even be raised against Nozick: Is it not that by going on strike, physicians are guilty of the same offence they level against the government or whatever organ responsible for their salaries and working conditions; that of being unjust to their patients and the public?

As has been seen, arguments by strike partisans are unsustainable and philosophically implausible. They are all narrow in that they look at strikes solely from an economic perspective. Yet, the question of strike is at root and indeed largely ethical, and not wholly an economic issue. Having put to rest arguments by pro-strike partisans as futile in solving the question on morality and legitimacy of physician strike, let us now turn to con-strike arguments – arguments which support the position of this book. It is the conviction of the paper that these arguments though need either refinement or reconstitution or both offer a solid answer to the question of the morality and legitimacy of physicians strike. The ensuing section shall therefore examine arguments against physicians; modify or reconstruct them where necessary in a bid to demonstrate how formidable arguments against physicians' strike are. Four arguments; argument based on a modified version of Hippocratic Oath, argument from the principle of beneficence, argument from utilitarianism and argument from African communalism shall be forwarded to reinforce the con-physician strike position.

The Con- Physician Strike View

Most of the con-strike partisans have forwarded arguments against physicians' strike based on the 'old version of the Hippocratic Oath'. For various reasons, as shall be seen, these arguments have been perceived as philosophically implausible and so have faced serious criticisms. For this reason, I shall defend the anti-physician strike view not only using a modified version of the Hippocratic Oath; but three arguments namely; argument from the principle of beneficence, argument from utilitarianism, and argument from African communalism.

Argument from Hippocratic Oath

Roth defines the Hippocratic Oath as an ethical perspective in ancient Greece which contends that the knowledge of medicine and that of medical ethics is available only to the Hippocratic physicians.[10] The Hippocratic physicians were a group of committed physicians (women and youth excluded) in ancient Greece who would use treatment to help the sick according to their ability and judgment but never with a view to injury and wrongdoing and, sometimes give their services for free.[11] The Oath stresses that only men, and not women can assume the duties of physicians. A number of questions can, however, be raised: Isn't it that women are naturally more loving and caring than men? And, don't we have some cases in the medical fraternity that require only women physicians, and not men to handle? It is in the light of these questions that the Hippocratic Oath and all arguments based on it have suffered criticism. And though a formidable challenge to the pro-physician strike partisans, all arguments based on it have been criticized for being sexist, selective, elitist and paternalistic. Having made these observations, the researcher of this work argue for the modification of the Hippocratic Oath to include both sexes and age groups (men and women, young and old) before advancing the argument that the Hippocratic Oath (the new version) can act as the source of power and reason for those who argue against physicians' strike. The Hippocratic Oath, thus, should be understood as an ethical perspective which contends that the knowledge of medicine and that of medical ethics is available to all physicians[12], men and women, young and old to...help the sick (sometimes free of charge) according to their (physicians) ability and judgment but never with a view to injury and wrongdoing[13]. Understood as such, this precept can be considered the heart of the ethical commitment shared by all physicians world-wide and it calls for mutual understanding and a high degree of collective responsibility on all physicians. It clearly acknowledges that physicians must reconcile two opposing orders-one based on the primacy of the covenant with patients and the other based on the ethos of self-interest. In this vein, physicians face the tension between self-interest and altruism, of which, to uphold self-interest by going on strike would turn them into entrepreneurs, businesspersons or agents of fiscal, social or economic policy. It is on the basis of this understanding that it can be argued that physicians (men and women, young and old) are morally obliged not to go on strike, but to display their special knowledge, skills and commitment to principles requiring the use of those skills altruistically. And this social mandate should be grounded at medical school. Otherwise, medicine will be expressed in a fatally distorted way; hence losing its originality and meaning. It can still be argued on the basis of the Hippocratic Oath that physicians in most if not all countries are trained for free using tax payers' money and government institution like national hospitals. Their knowledge, therefore, is not proprietary but acquired through the privilege of a medical education. This connotes that by accepting the privilege of a medical education, those who enter into medicine become parties to the Hippocratic Covenant with the society- one that cannot be dissolved unilaterally.[14] In other words, medical students, from their first day, enter into a community bound by a moral covenant; a covenant that calls for full responsibility of stewardship of medical knowledge they obtain at free price. Moreover, this covenant is acknowledged publicly when the physicians take an Oath at graduation.[15] The Oath is a public promise that the new physician understands the gravity of his or her calling and therefore promises to use competence in the interests of the sick and the public-fidelity to patients and the public. In this light, to argue that physicians should go on strike whenever they deem necessary is a violation of the covenant of trust and canons of medical ethics- a gross misunderstanding of the parameters and ethical principles that guide medicine in its proper functioning. In fact, strikes shrink physicians' professional latitude and diminish their professionalism as such.

Argument from the Principle of Beneficence

More commonly in biomedicine, beneficence is understood as a principle of medical ethics that requires that physicians benefit as well as prevent and remove harmful conditions from patients.[16] The principle has its source from the Hippocratic Oath. In the light of the definition of beneficence explicated above, I identify with Veatch who argues that: "Medicine is at heart a moral community and will always be; that those who practice it are 'de facto' members of a moral community bound together by knowledge and ethical precepts; and that, as a result, physicians have a collective as well as individual moral obligation to protect the welfare of sick persons.[17]" This is to say that physicians as a group of morally committed persons should always seek the greater balance of good over harm in the care of patients. An important question arises at this juncture: Does physicians' strike seeks the greater balance of good over harm in the care of patients? It is the conviction of this paper that this can never be. Actually, physicians strike does more harm than good, not only to the patients, but members of the public- it (strike) is in itself a crime against humanity committed by the physicians veneered by relentless pursuit of self-interest motives. This is not to say that physicians are not human beings with interests and needs alike other human beings. However they should understand that their profession is a calling- a serious de facto obligation which requires them to always seek the greater balance of good over harm in the care of patients. In subtle ways, the virtues of a good person and of the good physician overlap.[18] More importantly, it remains a truism that medicine as a profession and members of the public implicitly expect physicians to remain members of a moral community dedicated to altruism other than self-interest. To place self-interest ahead of the interests and needs of the patients would therefore mean converting the medical profession into a trade -a total abnegation of the very essence of what it means to be a physician. It is toleration of practical incompetence and selfish motives with incalculable long-term effects; hence is morally unjustifiable.

Argument from Utilitarianism

Utilitarianism is a doctrine which states that the rightness or wrongness of an action is determined by the goodness or badness of its consequences.[19] This means that utilitarianism is a consequentialist theory in so far as it calls for the assessment of actions in terms of their ends and consequences, their contribution to happiness and prevention of suffering. In fact, according to utilitarianism, an action is good or right when it achieves the greatest happiness for the greatest number, otherwise it is bad. Kantian ethics, based on the concept of duty, holds that an action is good if it is based on good intention. For utilitarians, an action in itself has no moral worth and takes moral value only when it is considered in conjunction with its effects. To the contrary, Kantians argue that what makes an action right is not its consequence(s) but the fact that it conforms to the moral law[20]. Thus unlike deontological theories which look at the action itself, utilitarianism assess the rightness or wrongness of an individual or group's action directly by its consequences and nothing else. De George offers some clarification of consequentialist and deontological ethics: "One approach argues on the basis of consequences (consequentialist); it states that whether an action is right or wrong depends on the consequences of that action. The second basic approach is called the deontological approach. It states that duty is the basic moral category, and that duty is independent of consequences. An action is right if it has certain characteristics or is of a certain kind, and wrong if it has other characteristics or is of a certain kind."[21] Utilitarianism and Kantian ethics are examples of consequentialist and deontological ethics, respectively. For Kant (the representative of Kantian ethics) the moral law or the highest principle of morality is based on human reason. This work does not seek to undertake a comprehensive discussion of consequentialist and deontological ethics, but to demonstrate the usefulness and plausibility of utilitarianism in criticizing physicians strike. However, any ethical theory that begins from some external demands and consequences faces the challenge of legitimacy. The challenge is that what ought to be done remains foreign to who ought to do it. Such an approach to ethics largely ignores the personality of the individual that guarantees the actions. Transposing the utilitarianism to physicians' strike, it is undoubtedly true that strike by physicians result in unbearable suffering of not only the patients in hospitals, but also of the public in general and the nation at large. During physicians' strike, unnecessary and premature deaths-deaths that could have been prevented are inevitable. According to IRINnews, during a 2008 strike by Zimbabwean physicians, Jestina Moyo of Bulawayo, expressed disappointment on arriving at Mpilo central hospital in Bulawayo, with her seriously ill son only to be told that doctors were on strike. She laments:

This is painful to watch my son waste away like this. The hospital says the doctors are on strike, demanding high

90

salaries, and there is nothing I can do for my son, as I have no money to take him to a private doctor. As it is, my son will die a painful death unless I find money to take him to a private doctor.[22]

According to the same source, since the strike started several death were registered which doctors could have dealt with if they were not on strike. The same consequences have been felt in other countries the world-over. In Malawi, for example, Kelita Kamoto, director of the Queen Elizabeth Central Hospital in Malawi's largest city Blantyre reported that between 15 and 20 deaths are recorded daily......deaths were registered as the strike entered its third week[23]. In another report by Ecumenical News International (ENI), Nigeria:

Constant strikes by Nigerian doctors this year are said to have claimed the lives of more than 20000 patients and have placed a massive burden on Christian hospitals across the country which have been overwhelmed with patients. And other 6000 accident victims died from lack of medical attention as a result of the doctors' strike.[24]

In Zambia, The Post Newspaper reported that:

Last month, nurses and doctors went on a month-long strike, forcing one Zambian mother to give birth on the sidewalk outside the University Teaching Hospital, the country's biggest. Her traumatized family took a picture of the ill-fated childbirth, showing the infant's legs stretching out of the mother, struggling for life -- the hospital and potential medical help tantalizingly nearby but completely out of reach. She gave birth without aid from doctors and the new-born died.[25]

Apart from Zimbabwe, Malawi, Nigeria and Zambia, in the past 20 years there has been strikes by medical doctors in Australia, Belgium, Canada, Chile, Finland, France, Germany, Ghana, India, Ireland, Israel, Italy, Korea, Malta, New Zealand, Peru, Serbia, Spain, Sri Lanka, Romania, USA and UK to name but a few. Many of these strikes have caused lasting damage from which health systems have struggled to get over; have been very costly (both in the short and long term); and have not achieved what the management appear to have wanted. It can also be argued on the basis of utilitarianism that physicians strike like that of the army, police and prison officers has far reaching consequences to the country in question; may result in violation of human rights and looting of public 'goods'. One can imagine what may happen if the army, police officers and the prison officers go on strike? If prison officers, for example, go on strike criminals, some with recorded history of mass killing will be free and obviously disturb the harmony of the innocent people. I believe physicians strike causes the same blow to the country involved. It is therefore the contention of this work that just like soldiers, prison officers and police officers who in many countries are not allowed to go on strike, physicians should likewise take no part in any form of strike action. In view of cases of unnecessary deaths and sufferings of both the patients and the public spelled out in this work, it is undeniable on the basis of utilitarianism that physicians strike has far reaching consequences not only to the patients, but to the public and the national government in question (to the majority). It has been exhibited that the happiness that physician strike brings is clearly overwhelmed by the suffering and sadness it causes to the majority (the patients, public and the government in question). From this understanding the paper contends that physicians strike can never be morally justifiable. Strike fails to achieve a greater happiness to the greatest number of people affected by it.

Argument from African Communalism

The African scholars surveyed, with the possible exception of Ghanaian philosopher Kwame Gyekye, regard African concepts of the individual and self to be almost totally dependent on and subordinate to social entities and cultural processes.[26] Kenyan theology professor John S. Mbiti, for example, believes that the individual has little latitude for self-determination outside the context of the traditional African family and community. He writes: "whatever happens to the individual happens to the whole group, and whatever happens to the whole group happens to the individual'. The individual can only say: 'I am, because we are; and since we are, therefore I am'; this is a cardinal point in the understanding of the African view of personhood."[27] Picking it from Mbiti's understanding, it is clear that the unnecessary suffering of the patients caused by physician strike does not only negatively affect the patients, but also the public and the physicians themselves as members of the group. Concurring with Mbiti, South African philosophy professor Augustine Shutte, cites the Xhosa proverb: *umuntu ngumuntu ngabantu* (a person is a person through persons). [28] He elaborates that: This (proverb) is the Xhosa expression of a notion that is common to all African languages and traditional cultures.[29] It cuts across all African cultures. For Ghanaian philosopher

Kwame Gyekye, the individual, although originating from and inextricably bound to his family and community, nevertheless possesses a clear concept of himself/herself as a distinct person of volition. It is from this combined sense of personhood and communal membership that the family and community expect individuals to take personally enhancing and socially responsible decisions and actions. Although he accepts that the dominant entity of African social order is the community, Gyekye believes:

It would be more correct to describe that order as amphibious, for it manifests features of both communality and individuality. African social thought seeks to avoid the excesses of the two exaggerated systems, while allowing for a meaningful, albeit uneasy, interaction between the individual and the society.[30]

Agreeing with Gyekye, Senegalese philosopher Leopold Senghor regards traditional African society to be based both on the community and on the person and in which, because it was founded on dialogue and reciprocity, the group had priority over the individual without crushing him, but allowing him to blossom as a person.[31] In the same stroke, Achebe commenting on Africa and Africans noted that Africa is not only a geographical expression; it is also a metaphysical landscape-it is in fact a view of the world and of the whole cosmos perceived from a particular position. Achebe goes further to argue that being an African is more than just a matter of passports or of individual volition[32] but of sensibility and responsibility. For Achebe and convincingly so being an African carries penalties. Okot P'Bitek picks up this argument and stresses that in African philosophy, man is not born free to do whatever he wants; in fact it is not even desirable to be so even if it were possible.[33] Thus persons are defined by reference to the environing community, not by focusing on this or that physical or psychological characteristics of the lone individual. This idea has been captured by other several African writers. Mbiti, for example, noted that the Africans' traditional view of person can be summed up in the statement "I am because we are and since we are, therefore I am."[34] One obvious conclusion to be drawn from this dictum is that personhood in the African traditional context is understood and defined by reference to other members of the same community. A person is defined through other members of his/her community. In this view, physicians in the African context are defined through members of their society (the patients and the public in general). They are physicians because of the people (patients and members of the public) they serve and are part. The relationship between physicians and other members of his/her community (patients and members of the public) can be represented by the syllogism: 1) an individual in the African society is defined through others; 2) A physician (in the African view point) is an individual who lives in a society. Therefore, a physician is defined through other members of his/her society. As spelled out above, the reality of the communal world takes precedence over the reality of individual life histories, whatever these may be. In the light of this, it is inescapably true that in the African context and indeed other contexts where people share the same idea of personhood and communal life, physician strike is violation of the public trust- a complete failure to exhibit the prime duty and responsibility to other members of their community. It is thus not only morally unjustifiable but also unfair and unjust to other members of the community. This is so because in any society (where people have the common goals) each member has his duties and responsibilities which s/he should accomplish with all the cogency, dedication and efficiency for his good and the good of the society. This connotes that an African is born with duties and responsibility to his society and the society in turn bestows rights and privileges on its members.[35] The values of individuals and individual rights, for example, are normally overridden by the values and rights of the community as a whole (to which the individual belongs).

Conclusion

One of the concerns of philosophers of medicine/medical ethicists has been to reflect on the rights, entitlements and obligation of physicians in relation to patients and members of the public. Scientists such as physicians inclined to dealing with factual judgments have failed to convincingly address the issue of strike using the "old version" of the Hippocratic Oath which is the bedrock of the medical profession the world over. Whilst the argument based on the 'new version' of the Hippocratic Oath, argument from the principle of beneficence, argument from utilitarianism, and argument from African communalism are philosophically plausible as has been demonstrated by this work, it is paramount to reiterate that the question of physician strike is too complex to be epitomized in a word. While there are shades of truth in each of the arguments raised in the prior discussion, they are all debatable. One can still argue that physician strikes are morally justifiable since physicians are people with families who need to be financially supported and cared for. Nevertheless, I remain supremely confident that physicians strike is always morally unjustifiable. Like Plato in The Republic, and like Aristotle, Aquinas and Dewey, I believe that physicians should through practice, by example, and by the study of ethics learn what it is to be a good physician qua physician, and to practice and value the virtues requisite for good medicine as I have spelled them out in this paper. If any problem, physicians should negotiate peacefully through their associations, courts of law, patients committees, moralists, academics and other stakeholders without contravening the virtues of medicine. They should convince the government or responsible authority for their salaries and conditions of services by arguments and not strike as the latter is detrimental not only to the government/responsible authority, but to patients and members of the public. It is therefore the contention of this paper that to argue that physicians strike is morally unjustifiable is not to say that physicians have no moral rights and entitlements. They do have as they are also human beings who feel, desire and need to be loved and respected by their fellow comrades. However, if problems arise with the employer these should be resolved amicably without losing the essential values of medicine by harming the society (which they are part). In fact, even if it means the revision of medicine's past to meet its future, this should be done without sacrificing their (physicians) traditional ethical values and causing harm to the patients and the public. By staging a strike the medical fraternity, thus, loses legitimacy and public confidence. After all, when striking the real people who suffer most are the patients and the public, and not the government or the body responsible for their plights and grievances. Physicians are indeed called to work for the people and strikes shrink their professional latitude and diminish them as professionals; hence the need to go back to tradition.

Notes

1. Strike action, accessed 22 June 2010. hptt://en.wikipedia.org.wiki/Talk:Strike action

2. Trade Union, accessed 22 June 2010. hptt://www.direct.gov.uk/en/Employment/TradeUnion/index.htm

3. Twentieth dynasty of Egypt, accessed 22 June 2010. http://en.wikipedia.org/wiki/Twentieth_dynasty_of_Egypt

4. Beauchamp TL, Childress JF. *Principles of Biomedical Ethics*, Oxford. Oxford University Press, 1989:256

5. Beauchamp TL, Childress JF.3rd Ed. *Principles of Biomedical Ethics*, Oxford. Oxford University Press, 1989, p. 254-255.

6. Pellegrino E, Thomasma DC. *The Virtues in Medical Practice*, New York. Oxford University Press, 1993, p.92.

7. Rawls J.A. 'Theory of Justice', in Boss AJ. Ed, *Perspectives on Ethics*, London. Mayfield Publishing Company, 1998, p.351.

8. Rawls J.A Theory of Justice, in Boss AJ. Ed, *Perspectives on Ethics*, London. Mayfield Publishing Company, 1998, p.352.

9. Nozick R. Anarchy, *State and Utopia*, New York. Basic Books, 1974, p.150.

10. Roth BR. 'Medicine's Ethical Responsibilities' In Veatch RM. Ed, *Cross Cultural Perspective in Medical Ethics*, Jones and Bartlett Publishers,1989, p.149.

11. Jones WHS. Trans. *Hippocrates*, Harvard: Harvard University Press, 1923, p.1947.

12. Roth BR. Medicine's Ethical Responsibilities in Veatch RM. Ed, *Cross Cultural Perspective in Medical Ethics*, Jones and Bartlett Publishers,1989, p.148-149.

13. Jones WHS. Trans. Hippocrates, Harvard. Harvard University Press, 1923:1947-148

14. Beauchamp TL, Childress JF. *Principles of Biomedical Ethics, Oxford.* Oxford University Press, 1989, p.32.

15. Beauchamp TL, Childress JF. *Principles of Biomedical Ethics*, Oxford. Oxford University Press, 1984, p.32-33.

16. Beauchamp TL, Childress JF. *Principles of Biomedical Ethics*, Oxford. Oxford University Press, 1984, p.13.

17. Veatch RM. Ed, *Cross Cultural Perspective in Medical Ethics*, Jones and Bartlett Publishers, 1989.

18. Pellegrino E, Thomasma DC. *The Virtues in Medical Practice*, New York. Oxford University Press, 1993, p.176.

19. Smart JJC. 'Utilitarianism,' In *Encyclopaedia of Philosophy*, Macmillan. London, 1996, p.206.

20. De George RT, Business Ethics, New York. Macmillan Publishing Company, 1982, p.58.

21. De George RT, *Business Ethics*, New York: Macmillan Publishing Company, 1982, p.37.

22. Zimbabwe: Doctors' strike adds to country's pain, IRINnews, 26 August 2008. Available online @ *http://www.irinnews.org/*

23. More TB Patients Die due to Doctors Strike in Malawi, 14 October 2001. Available online@*http://www.highbeam.com/Xinhua+News+Agency/publications.aspx?date=2001Q4.*

24. Nigeria's Doctors' Strike Leaves Christian Hospitals Inundated, Ecumenical News International. 25 February 2005. Available online @ *http://www.eni.ch*.

25. 'Zambian woman forced to have child without medical help, baby dies!', 20 November 2009. *The Post*, Lusaka: Zambia. Available online @

http://www.netmums/coffeehouse/general-chat-514/new-current-affairs-topical discussion-12/308587-zamian-womam-forced-havechild-without-medical-help-baby-dies.html

26. Gyekye K. *The Unexamined Life: Philosophy and the African Experience*, Accra. Ghana Universities Press, 1988.

27. Mbiti, J.S. *African Religions and Philosophy*, New York. Praeger Publishers, 1969, p.109.

28. Shutte, A. *Philosophy for Africa, South Africa.* University of Cape Town Press, 1993, p.46-47.

29. Shutte, A. *Philosophy for Africa, South Africa.* University of Cape Town Press, 1993, p. 47-48.

30. Gyekye K. The Unexamined Life: Philosophy and the African Experience, Accra. Ghana Universities Press, 1988: 31-32.

31. Senghor L. 'Negritude and African Socialism', St. Anthony's Papers. London. Oxford University Press, 1963; 3(1): 16-22.

32. Achebe, C. *Hopes and Impediments*, New York. Anchor Books, 1990, p.17.

33. P'Bitek O. In Wiredu, K. *A Critique of Western Scholarship on African Religion*, Wiley-Blackwell, 2005.

34. Mbiti, J.S. *African Religions and Philosophy*, New York. Praeger Publishers, 1969, p.145.

35. Mawere, M. 'On Pursuit of the Purpose Life: The Shona Metaphysical Perspective,' *Journal of Pan African Studies.* 2010; 3 (6):269-284.

Chapter Six

Advertising in African Traditional Medicine

This chapter critically examines the morality of advertising by practitioners in spiritual healing and herbal medicine heretofore referred to as traditional medicine, in southern African urban societies. While the subject of traditional medicine has been heavily contested in medical studies in the last few decades, the monumental studies on the subject have emphasised the place of traditional medicine in basic health services. Insignificant attention has been devoted to examine the ethical problems associated with traditional medicine advertising. Critical look at the worthiness of some advertising strategies used by has been largely ignored. Yet, though advertising is key to helping traditional medicine practitioners' products and services known by prospective customers, this research registers a number of morally negative effects that seem to outweigh the merits that the activity brings to prospective customers. The work adopts southern African urban societies, and in particular Mozambique, South Africa and Zimbabwe as particular references. The choice of the trio is not accidental, but based on the fact that these countries have in the last few decades been flooded with traditional medicine practitioners/traditional healers from within the continent and from abroad. Most of these practitioners use immoral advertising strategies in communicating to the public the products and services they offer. It is against this background that this work examines the morality of advertising strategies deployed by practitioners in launching their products and services. To examine the moral worthiness of the advertising strategies used by traditional medical practitioners, I used qualitative analysis of street adverts as well as electronic and print media. From the results obtained through thematic content analysis, the work concludes that most of the practitioners in traditional medicine lack both business and medical ethics. That said, the work urges practitioners to seriously consider the morality of their adverts as in most cases they (adverts) do more harm than good. Further to that, it (the work) recommends the governments of the affected countries to put in place stringent measures to address this mounting problem.

Background to Traditional Medicine Advertising

Healthy has always been a concern for all human societies since the beginning of history. In the Western world traditional medicine dates back to ancient Greece and its famous doctors like Hippocrates and Galen. However, although all other civilizations from the ancient world were using plants as natural remedies for their ailments the first documented accounts of the use of herbs as traditional medicine originated in China.[1] In African societies and in Asia in general, though traditional medicine has been used for centuries now, its use seems to have increased in the contemporary times with the advent of diseases like HIV/Aids.

In the African continent, Mozambique, South Africa and Zimbabwe are some of the countries in the fore on the use of traditional medicine. In these countries, socio-economic and political pressures in addition to the prevalence of deadly diseases such as HIV/Aids contribute to the use of traditional medicine. This is to say that the use of traditional medicine has reached an advanced stage in southern Africa in the last few decades mainly through medical traditional practitioners/traditional healers. Having made the same observation, Olapade notes that there has been a global resurgence in traditional medicine in the last ten years probably because of many of the known synthetic drugs in allopathic or Western medicines for the treatment of various ailments are failing or that the causes of these various diseases are developing resistance to the known drugs.[2]

Besides, in southern African societies like Mozambique, South Africa and Zimbabwe traditional medicine healing has been associated with witchcraft, hence viewed with negative and pejorative connotations. This has been chiefly because of Eurocentric paradigms of Africa where the perjured interpretations of Africa have remained grafted on the mental processes and human aspirations of modern Africans thereby robbing them of their intellectual confidence and mental identities with regard to posterity. Unfortunately, many traditional medicine practitioners have stretched this kind of thinking further through their immoral advertising strategies.

However, as previously highlighted the massive socio-cultural, economic and political changes in southern Africa since the attainment of political independence have generated immense pressure on the post-colonial states to provide primary health care for all. These changes have brought in renewed socio-economic challenges in the region. Consequently, many people have resorted to traditional medicine; "the role and efficacy of traditional medicine and spiritual services have once again moved to the spotlight."[3] These courses of events explain the reason why a new crop of traditional medicine practitioners from different countries in the region has emerged claiming to be well-researched, gifted and educated. It has been estimated by Ritcher that in South Africa, for example, between 60% and 80% of the population currently rely on the traditional medical sector as their first contact for advice and treatment of health concerns.[4] Such an increased demand in traditional medicine services in the region (southern Africa) has lured not only practitioners from within the region, but from as far as India and China. Thus, there has been increased competition among traditional medicine practitioners, leading them to employ all advertising tactics and strategies at their disposal in order to lure customers and withstand the fierce competition from other practitioners. Most if not all of these practitioners have therefore been caught up in ethical quandaries-moral dilemmas- on how they should advertise themselves in a way that would make them more popular than others. From the results obtained from this study, it appears that most of the practitioners have decided to shun "clean advertising" or acceptable moral advertising strategies in favour of "dirty advertising," that is, immoral advertising strategies. This is chiefly because it has not been easy for most of the practitioners to withstand competition from their counterparts. In the light of this situation, the drive for profit making seems to be overriding many traditional healers' ought to be morally upright. Thus, the upsurge of immoral business practices in urban southern African societies is testimonial to the unwillingness of the privies to these social ills. So is the prevalence of the so-called myth of amoral business that has invaded the traditional medicine arena.

That said, this chapter examines the interface of advertising strategies and morality/ethics in the context of traditional medicine in southern African urban societies. For purposes of this work, the concept morality shall be used interchangeably with ethics. Using qualitative analysis of selected cases of adverts drawn from the aforementioned countries of reference's street corners, electronic and print media, I argue that the persuasive techniques that are employed in advertising by those in traditional medicine often do more harm (to prospective customers) than good. While in business, adverts are meant to truthfully inform the public/prospective customers about the goods and services that are available on the market, those by the practitioners in southern African urban societies normally say the opposite of the reality on the ground.

In view of the foregoing, this book argues for the integration of business and ethics from two main dimensions namely African communalism, utilitarianism and or consequentialist approach. Using these dimensions, the relationship between business elements like advertising and practitioners in traditional medicine is examined.

Although it is acknowledged in this work that the answer to medicinal business- moral problems is very difficult to stipulate, it is suggested in this book that moral teaching, through civic education to the public (potential customers/consumers) and the traditional healers is necessary. Overall, this chapter makes an attempt to reconstruct and integrate an ethical culture in traditional medicine by demonstrating how the deployment of some advertising techniques by some traditional healers flout the basic principles of both medical and business ethics.

Conceptual Analysis of Herbal medicine, spiritual healing and/or traditional medicine

Since previously noted the present chapter critically examines the morality of advertising by practitioners in spiritual healing and herbal medicine, also referred to as traditional medicine, there is need to define herbal medicine and spiritual healing before looking at the history of advertising practices in modern Africa. Herbal medicine and spiritual healing have not been easy concepts to define with precision. However, technical definitions have been offered. According to Australian Journal of Herbalism (http://www.nhaa.org.au/index.php?) herbal medicine is medicine made exclusively from plants; it refers to using a plant's seeds, berries, roots, leaves, bark, or flowers for medicinal purposes.[5] It is the oldest and still the most widely used system of medicine outside of conventional medicine in all cultures in the world today. It is important to note that herbal medicine is also known as botanical medicine or phytomedicine which means using a plant's seeds, berries, roots, leaves, bark, or flowers for medicinal purposes.[6] As given by the same source, herbal medicine is becoming more mainstream as improvements in analysis and quality control along with advances in clinical research show the value of herbal medicine in the treating and preventing disease. However, scientists are still unsure of what specific ingredient in a particular herb works to treat a condition or illness. This is because the whole herbs contain many ingredients, and they may work together to produce a beneficial effect. Many factors determine how effective an herb will be. For example, the type of environment (climate, bugs, soil quality) in which a plant grew will affect it, as will how and when it was harvested and processed.[7]

While herbal medicine is somehow technically easy to define, spiritual healing is not. According to Grayson most people think of spiritual healing as faith healing, but it is not.[8] For him, faith healing has to do with an unquestioned belief in some great God "out there" or some vast power — also "out there". Sometimes it takes the form of a shaman, a person who is empowered to produce extraordinary, magical effects in the world of the person who believes in him. These aspects explain why the definition of spiritual healing difficult to pin down with precision, therefore contentious. However Grayson notes that the underlying principle of spiritual healing is that in the spiritual mind healing process, one does not deal with unquestioned belief in any holy person, religious rite, sacred place or object. Instead, one deals directly with the truth of being which should be perceived metaphysically as part of the underlying Reality of Life. During spiritual healing, the metaphysical inner patterns of consciousness inevitably appear as an outer world of experience, thereby making one conscious of the truth that life belongs to God, or the Great Spirit. It is this realization that enables one to perform spiritual healing.

Critical analysis of definitions of herbal medicine and spiritual healing above shows a broad range of characteristics and elements that make the two interwoven and therefore hardly distinguished from each other. As such, there has been no standard definition for spiritual healing[9] and herbal medicine as both terms can refer to widely varying practices, and there are many ways in which they overlap. It is for this reason and for purposes of this work, that both the term spiritual healing and herbal medicine are used to refer to traditional medicine. That said, we also need to define traditional medicine. World Health Organization's (WHO) definition of traditional medicine which says:

Traditional medicine includes diverse health practices, approaches, knowledge and beliefs incorporating plant, animal and/or mineral based medicines, spiritual therapies, manual techniques and exercises applied singularly or in combination to maintain well-being, as well as to treat, diagnose or prevent illness.[10]

As has been highlighted above, in Africa and as elsewhere, herbal medicine and spiritual healing are both embodied within traditional medicine which in itself is the total sum of all knowledge and practices used by traditional healers in diagnosis, prevention and elimination of physical, mental or societal imbalance. This knowledge or practices can be explicable or not. The underlying fact is the knowledge/practices are handed down spontaneously from one generation to another, normally through the aid of a traditional medicine practitioner/traditional healer. This can be through orature, literature, observation or even through mystical ways. I identify with Pretorius who defines traditional medicine practitioner/traditional healer is defined as:

Someone who is recognized by the community in which he lives as competent to provide health care by using vegetable, animal substances and certain other methods based on social, cultural and religious backgrounds as well as the prevailing knowledge, attitudes and beliefs regarding physical, mental and social- well-being and the causation of disease and disability in the community.[11]

As already alluded to above, there are two main kinds of traditional healers that can be identified. These are identified by Ritcher as: herbalists and diviners (diagnostician or divine mediums respectively).[12] It should however be noted that different ethnic groups have their own legends about the origins of traditional medicine in their own society.

Advertising in traditional medicine in sub-Saharan Africa

Sub-Saharan Africa has a long tradition of traditional medicine advertising. In the past, advertising was normally done orally, that is, by word of mouth. This was done by the practitioners themselves and or by clients and neighbours. As such, advertising of traditional medicine though now more common than ever is not a new and unique phenomenon to southern Africa, but is resonant as in other countries in the region and beyond.

While the subject of traditional medicine has been heavily contested in medical studies by Offiong, for example, in the last few decades in sub-Saharan countries like the abovementioned the monumental studies on these subjects[13] have emphasised the place of traditional medicine in basic health service. Adegoju though have criticized the abovementioned scholars has fallen in the same trap as he takes a linguistic stance and focuses solely on the rhetorical style used by herbal medical practitioners in South-western Nigeria in launching their products[14]. As such, all the aforementioned scholars, among others, have devoted insignificant or no attention to examining the moral worthiness of some advertising strategies used by practitioners in traditional medicine when launching their products and services on market. Yet, though advertising is key to helping practitioners' products and services known by prospective customers, this research establishes a number of morally negative effects that seem to outweigh the merits that the activity brings to society.

In urban societies of Mozambique, South Africa and Zimbabwe, the linguistic advertising strategies employed by traditional medicine practitioners/traditional healers have mired the advertising of herbal and spiritual healing services with a plethora of controversies. The controversies are further compounded by the nature of advertising discourse itself which many business ethicists like R.T. DeGeorge[15] and Munyaradzi Mawere in his 2010 publication believe is psychologically coercing, misinforming, cunning and void of ethical principles.

In addition, though Mozambique, South Africa and Zimbabwe are some of the countries with a very long history of the development and use of herbal medicine and spiritual healing techniques, the national governments of these countries have always suppressed traditional medicine's advertising and use in favour of conventional/scientific medicine. This is because traditional medicine has always been associated with witchcraft. It should be noted that in these countries colonial systems' health care legacy remains a problem with their bias towards allopathic health care. In fact the debate on the legitimacy of traditional healers has been highly contentious because of the complex political, legal, cultural and social ramifications of the practice. From a politico-historical perspective, the colonial government regimes perplexed by failure to establish and provide proof and distinction between traditional healing and witchcraft in legal battles outlawed both [traditional healing and witchcraft] for legal and administrative convenience. Unsurprisingly, the post southern African governments haunted by the same dilemma retained the colonial legislations like the Witchcraft Suppression Act where formal courts of law were under obligation not to recognize both traditional healing practices and witchcraft unless the plaintiff provided substantial evidence linking the defendant to the practice. In Zimbabwe, for example, this saw the enactment of the Zimbabwe's Witchcraft Suppression Act (ZWSA) (Chapter 73) which considers as illegal an activity that has to do with supernatural forces or charm meant to inflict injury, misfortunes, illness or death. Likewise, South Africa saw the enactment of restrictive legislations such as the Witchcraft Suppression Act in 1957 and the Witchcraft Suppression Amendment Act of 1970. In Mozambique, though no known laws were enacted against witchcraft or activities related to it, traditional healing until recently was equated to witchcraft. Worse still and in line with the misplaced thinking against traditional medicine practitioners (as elsewhere in the region), there have been numerous media reports about people who have been killed for *muti* (charm used in witchcraft) purposes under the instruction of traditional practitioners. As Mutungi puts it:

Witchcraft beliefs embrace a wide range of ideas, practices, and motivations, but in their various forms they usually share the idea that the power to inflict injury and benefit could be exercised through unobservable, supernatural means.[16]

111

In southern Africa, the word witchcraft as the concept of traditional medicine has therefore earned negative and pejorative labels. This has been chiefly because of Eurocentric paradigms of Africa where the perjured interpretations of Africa have remained grafted on the mental processes and human aspirations of modern Africans thereby robbing them of their intellectual confidence and mental identities with regard to posterity. Unfortunately, many traditional medicine practitioners, especially those in contemporary urban societies have stretched further and authenticated this misplaced thinking through their immoral advertising strategies.

In the aforementioned countries, and sub-Sahara in general, the massive socio-cultural, economic and political changes since the attainment of political independence and a general renewed challenge to the post-colonial state to provide primary health care for all brought cultural crunches and challenges in the region. They [southern African states] had to resort to herbal medicine and spiritual healing, hence making "the role and efficacy of traditional medicine services once again moved to the spotlight."[17] These courses of events explain the reason why a new crop of traditional medicine practitioners from different countries in the region has emerged claiming, through advertising, to be well-researched, gifted and educated. It has been estimated that between 60% and 80% of South Africans currently rely on the traditional medical sector as their first contact for advice and treatment of health concerns.[18]

Due to socio-economic and political pressures in the southern African region, there has been increased demand in traditional medicine services luring not only practitioners from within the region, but from as far as India and China.

As a matter of consequence, there has been increased competition among traditional medicine practitioners, leading them to employ all tactics and strategies at their disposal. These include immoral advertising strategies like false testimonials and misinformation in order to lure customers and withstand the fierce competition from other service providers. As previously highlighted, most if not all of these practitioners have therefore tended to shun "clean advertising" in favour of "dirty advertising" in order to withstand competition from their counterparts. As never been before (in the past) profit making has emerged to challenge and override many traditional healers' ought to be morally upright. Thus, the upsurge of immoral business practices, through immoral advertising strategies, in contemporary southern African urban societies has reached an alarming level. So is the prevalence of the so-called myth of amoral business that has invaded the traditional medicine arena. Most traditional healers, for example, have generally accepted the myth of amoral business- "a belief that business and ethics do not mix"[19] -they are mortal enemies. They have done so by employing unscrupulous advertising tactics/strategies. Some of the unethical advertising practices that have unapologetically infiltrated the southern African herbal medicine and spiritual healing arenas are misinforming, coercing, cunning, deception and other such problems associated with advertising. These practices have manifested at an increasingly alarming rate invoking the anti- advertising partisans and the consumers in general arguing for the banning of advertising of traditional medicine by traditional healers.

What most if not all of these practitioners have forgotten or failed to realize is the fact that "dirty advertising"-immoral advertising strategies- void of acceptable ethical practices can dramatically compromise their reputation in the society. The deployment of "dirty advertising" has therefore presented a serious moral test case for traditional healers in traditional medicine in southern Africa and beyond.

Ethical Questions and Methodological Issues in Traditional Medicine

The present study seeks to address the questions: Which moral wrongs are being committed in the name of advertising by practitioners in traditional medicine? How best can we right the wrongs committed by practitioners in traditional medicine? As a researcher on medical issues on Africa in general and southern African region in particular, I have come to the realization that most researchers on traditional medicine such as Offiong (1999) and Iroegbu[20] have emphasised the place of herbal medicine in basic health service. Adegoju taking a linguistic stance, emphasizes on the rhetorical style used by traditional medicine practitioners in South-western Nigeria in launching their products.[21] All these scholars, among others, are guilt of devoting insignificant or no attention to examining the moral worthiness of some advertising strategies being used by practitioners in traditional medicine when launching their products and services on market. The history of traditional medicine thus makes a sorry reading with its failure to document, by default or otherwise, the moral wrongs committed in the name of advertising by practitioners in traditional medicine. The consequence is that these moral wrongs are perpetuated in societies thereby making the society suffering undeservingly; hence the need for a study as this.

As part of my research design, I relied on qualitative analysis of data sampled from both the electronic and print media. For the electronic media, I focused on jingles on television and radio in the three countries previously referred to. In addition to the jingles, I qualitatively focused on the thematic content of the specially sponsored programmes where the advertisers buy airtime that covers at least ten minutes slot or more. Such programmes normally involve interviews where the advertisers tell the audiences what they offer and sometimes the advertisers answer questions from the audiences. The jingles and sponsored programmes are drawn from radio and television stations based in the aforementioned cities. Jingles and sponsored programmes from these different cities were considered in order to come up with an unbiased view of adverts by most spiritual and herbal practitioners in southern African region. One striking observation on the advertisers sampled said more than what their medicines practically cure. Others directly or indirectly undermined conventional medicines thereby widening the gap between scientific medicine and traditional medicine.

The data sampled from print media were adverts and select paid by traditional medicine advertisers, mainly to newspapers, in the countries under study, that is, Mozambique, South Africa and Zimbabwe. It is important to note, however, that there is an overlap between adverts in electronic and print media.

In both electronic and print media, diseases and conditions commonly advertised by practitioners in traditional medicine were asthma, tuberculosis, matrimonial or love related problems, misfortune related problems, sexually transmitted diseases, sterility, low sperm count, among others.

To supplement the field observation information obtained from electronic and print media, the researcher used observation in the big cities of Mozambique, South Africa and Zimbabwe. The cities observed were Maputo, Beira (Mozambique), Johannesburg, Cape Town (South Africa) and Harare (Zimbabwe). A striking observation about the streets of these cities, where the researcher lived, studied and worked for some years, is the amount of pavement advertisements of traditional medicine services, mainly in the form of leaflets at strategic locations such as road sides, street corners, markets and motor parks where the attention of passers-by can easily be attracted. Using observation data collection procedure the researcher observed 45 pavement advertisements (6 in Beira; 9 in Maputo; 6 in Johannesburg; 9 in Cape Town and 15 in Harare) by different traditional medicine practitioners. The field observation, a method which the researcher adopted from his anthropological studies was used as one of the major collection tools to ascertain the project location and what really is happening on the ground. Observation allows the researcher to have access to first-hand information that s/he can observe and record in person. Using this method, the researcher observed that to reach their prospective customers, the advertisers issue out to passers or stick on corner posts leaflets detailing out the title(s), name(s), contact details and place of origin of the traditional healer and the available treatment services for various health ailments and socio-cultural and financial problems. This type of advertising is very aggressive and reaches out to the people directly.

Common Advertising Moral Wrongs in Traditional Medicine in Southern Africa

Business in all spheres, medical fraternity included, is bound by some precepts that all practitioners are obliged to observe. According to Fieser businesses have moral obligations beyond what the law sometimes requires.[22] This is to say "business is supposed to be unscrupulous and driven by the sole need for personal success. In other words, business should consider the customers' values, interests and needs."[23] This is contrary to what is transpiring in the advertisement of traditional medicine in southern African urban societies. Instead of what Fieser[24] proposes above, advertisement of herbal medicine and spiritual healing services is characterized by a plethora of moral wrongs. These range from psychological coercion, misinforming, exaggerated competence, false guarantees, and false testimonials to the use of rhetoric. Such practices flout and dramatically compromise the basic principles of both business and medical ethics and traditional healers' reputation in the society. In what follows, a detailed account of advertising moral wrongs abound in southern African societies is presented. Suggestions to deal with them are also given in the account.

Exaggerated Competence

The advertisement of traditional medicine in southern African societies has been characterized by the moral wrong of exaggerated competence. This is whereby the healer claims to cure diseases or heal problems of all kinds when in reality s/he doesn't have the power or knowledge to do so. This makes exaggerated competence a persuasive strategy that is employed in advertising traditional medicine to raise the healer's profile, credibility and competence. In such immoral advertising strategies, the advertisers pretend to be credible by displaying practical intelligence and in-depth knowledge of medicines and/or spiritual powers. The advertisers normally propagate this credibility in the eyes of prospective customers by clearly outlining the clinical symptoms of diseases, with the view of showing the public that they have thorough knowledge of pathology and could diagnose the patient's diseases even before interacting with them. Below are some of the adverts sampled in southern African urban societies during this study:

i) Abnormal Ejaculation?: Are you a "1minute man" get ejaculatory powder for you not to sperm quick that your women in stable relationship

ii) Diminished libido/sex drive?: Libido enhancer to give you strong urge in stable relationships.

iii) Erectile dysfunction?: This may be due to aging, diabetes, relationship stress hormones or physical problems. A new Herbal Chinese mixture it takes 20min before sex to give you rock hard erection permanently.

iv) Penis Pro-Enlarger: Have you failed from pills, creams, surgeries, pumps and false promises come try the new Chinese remedy & gel rubbed 2x daily for 1 week to the big cock you ever desired.

v) After fifteen years of thorough research, Prof. Dr. J.J. Diriko finally came to a breakthrough, now introducing (MASAI GEL) for the first time in Mozambique, especially for both men and women. It is a herbal gel from the MASAI land mainly Intended to enlarge the penis both in girth and length. In women the gel is prepared in such a manner that it causes the vagina to shrink thereby making a woman appearing a virgin in her late fifties.

The thematic contents of all these adverts undermine the strength of conventional medicine by emphasizing exaggerated competence of the Chinese herbs over scientific medicine. By providing a false detailed background information about oneself as is in the case of "Professor Dr. Diriko" the practitioner obviously intend to magnify his/her credibility. One would think that the healer is a well-educated, thorough and highly experienced person when in actual fact he has never attained any Doctoral degree, worse still Professorship. Also, making reference to the countries from which the mixtures, creams, gel and powders are sourced such as China, the advertisers make a gaze towards convincing prospective customers that their medicines are authentic as they come from countries which are well-known for producing effective herbal medicines. All these claims tend to underscore the herbal practitioners' insatiable quest for acceptability and credibility directed towards convincing or winning the minds of prospective customers. As such, adverts of this nature result in psychological coercion on the part of prospective customers who sometimes will have exhausted the use of scientific medicine.

What remains a truism is that no evidence can be practically made available to support such claims as those made above. In other words, no empirical or scientific evidence to prove that the advertised treatment will result in permanent healing without side effects or allergies is made available to prospective customers. Worse still, there is no evidence for the audience to prove that the healer can cure a myriad of diseases and conditions. It is in the face of this uneasiness that one can critically questions the moral acceptability of such claims. This work therefore advances the argument that by making exaggerated competence, the healer does not only transgress against the moral precept of advertisement which stresses truth, but compromise his/her moral legitimacy in the society. Also, the advert violates Gricean's maxim of quality, which states that in conversation (and by extension in advertising discourse) one should not lie or make unsupported claims.[25] Hence, affected people are encouraged to take their courage to denounce such adverts. This will serve as a moral whip to discipline and discourage advertisers of traditional medicine from engaging in such immoral advertising strategies as exaggerated competence.

False Guarantees

From the sampled data, it was also revealed through qualitative analysis of thematic content of some adverts that another advertising strategy being employed by advertisers of traditional medicine and spiritual healing is false guarantee. This advertising wrong is a persuasive technique which is meant to induce confidence in the potential customers most of whom are likely to have experienced the technique in the orthodox commercial world. It was observed that in southern African urban societies, false guarantees come in the form of false promises to prospective customers. The promises obtained from sampled data were:

i) Get back your lost property, relative or lover is less than two days after treatment.

120

ii) Call and book an appointment before you come in, the Dr is always busy.

iii) A distinguished miracle teller who tells who tells you all about your problems before you say anything and heals diseases of all kind.

iv) Just come in and do away with all your problems immediate after treatment. 100% guaranteed permanent results.

v) Excellent herbs with no side effects for all STDs, itching vagina, womb cleaning.

vi) ABORTION: Same day, 100% safe and pain free guaranteed. Call Dr. Donald.

The above guarantees raise a lot of questions, especially to critical thinkers though they [guarantees] are likely to convince prospective customers haunted by some of the problems outlined. The short time frame (of two days) guarantee, 100% guaranteed permanent results and promises to meet a distinguished miracle teller and restorer of lost properties are all false guarantees that have the potential to psychologically compel prospective customers to come in their numbers. However, on subjecting all these claims on hyperbole literary analysis one may realize that there is no authenticity in them; they are just hyperbole exaggerations used in the name of advertising to lure prospective customers by evoking their feelings. Hyperbole refers to a case where the speaker's description is stronger than is warranted by the state of affairs described.[26] It is from this understanding that I advance the argument that adverts by healers can only be morally justifiable in as long as they uphold truth and abandon the use of false guarantees and other such advertising gimmicks. In this view, I identify with Harris and

Seldon who understand advertising as "a form of communication designed to spread accurate information to the public with the view of promoting marketable goods and services."[27]

Misinformation

It is a generally well known adage that "lies when documented resemble truths". Having realized the impact of 'well cooked' and documented lies, most southern African advertisers in traditional medicine document eye catching inscriptions, catchy rhetorical titles and exaggerated achievements to win the hearts of their targeted audiences. Most of the titles sampled from southern African urban street corners, electronic and print media were: Prof Dr; Mama; Dr of the year; Best Prophet of all times; Magic man from the Pacific; Expert prince from Indian ocean; The Proud Winner of sub-Saharan Spiritual Healers Award; A well-educated, thorough going researcher; A distinguished miracle teller; A specialist of all spiritual problems; and the 2011 African herbalist winner.

Such rhetorical titles are used to create credibility and acceptance by the targeted audience, that is, prospective customers. By using such titles as above, the traditional medicine practitioners attempt to draw parallels between themselves and competent practitioners in conventional medicine who can be entrusted with human life. This confers legitimacy on the healers as the titles suggest that the bearer is competent, rigorous, educated and with formal training in the diagnosis and treatment of health-related ailments, usually in medical schools. What makes their claims dubious, especially to critics is however the fact that unlike mainstream medical

122

doctors who indicate their educational qualifications and the institutions from which they acquired them, practitioners under study don't do the same. This makes people understand that they are being deliberately misinformed. Yet, in an advertising pursuit, misinformation is a moral transgression against the public. Denouncing the immorality of misinformation, Norris argues that "the advertiser should always tell the whole truth about the product he wants to sell and should judge the message not by what it says but by what the reader is most likely to think it says."[28] The advertiser thus, should not manipulate, misinform or influence the prospective consumer deliberately or otherwise. The consumer should decide on his/her own without any physical or psychological coercion.

False Testimonials and claims of sources of herbs

The last advertising gimmick sampled in southern African urban societies during this study was the use of false testimonials and claims of sources of herbs. Testimonies by people who claim to have been healed by the practitioners were observed in contents of street corner adverts, electronic and print media. Far reaching sources of herbs were also given. The motivation behind the deployment of testimonies and mentioning far reaching sources of herbs is to create legitimacy, credibility and to instil confidence in prospective customers. It was observed that the people who give these testimonies normally provide their personal names and most of them were from low density suburbs. This was possibly meant to create the impression that the 'poor' prospective customers can also end up living in low density suburbs if they visit the practitioner. The sources of the herbs were also mainly under oceans/seas, famous mountains and sacred places. The strategy here thus is twofold: to make prospective customers believe that their problems can really be solved and that their lives can be improved just like those in the low density suburbs. Below are examples of testimonies and sources of herbs from the sampled data:

i) Having consulted several traditional healers but all disappointing me, I went to Dr. Diriko who helped me with magic stick. I now solved my financial problems. (Tatenda Mariyawanda, Borrowdale: Harare)

ii) My penis was small. I was shy to propose love to women! I was scared they will laugh at me. I used Chinese herb remedies and in less than 5 days my penis grew to the size I wanted (Peter Jones, Centurion: Pretoria)

iii) I always wanted to start my own business but in vain. When I met Dr. Pedro Domingos I picked a bundle of one thousand meticais by the roadside and started my business right away. I am a successful business man in T3 (Paulo Emanuel, Maputo)

iv) Dr. Abu Dimao with magical herbs from the Indian Ocean, Mount Kilimanjaro and the Kalahari desert.

v) Mama Dorina with spiritual powers and Chinese, Indian, African, American and Arabic herbs that heal over 100 diseases.

It should be noted that the claims of sources of herbs that are sacred, far and the use of testimonies with names of people healed are just but false. One would concur that if these claims and testimonies were true, nothing bad would be said about them. What raises concern is that from the sampled data, it was revealed that most of the names in the testimonies are inexistent. This was credibly true as during the study, the researcher never met any one of the people who made the testimonies; none of them ever came to the fore to show up himself/herself in the public. This has rendered all the sampled testimonies a gimmick and empty diplomacy deployed to engender confidence in prospective customers by raising their hopes. This advertising technique is well documented in the general advertising discourse and is known for invoking a propaganda technique called 'bandwagon'. Bandwagon is an attempt to persuade the targeted audience to join in and take the course of action that everyone else in a similar predicament is taking regardless of one's financial, health and social condition. The key aspect of testimonies is that they show prospective customers the benefits that other people are getting from healers.

The claim of supremacy over other healers or herbalists by practitioners under study is another false type of false testimony with the potential to make prospective customers believe that the healer in question is better than the rest. In philosophy circles, in particular logic, this technique is known as *fallacy-argumentum ad hominem*. This is a situation whereby people try to win arguments by saying derogatory and negative things about their opponents as is demonstrated in the adverts i) and ii) above. In advertising, this technique though immoral is normally used to out-compete one's counterparts, in this case, other spiritual and herbal medicine practitioners. It is in this light that I argue against false testimonials and false claims of sources of herbs used by most of the practitioners in traditional medicine in southern African urban societies.

Conclusion

In this chapter, it has been revealed that in contemporary southern African urban societies, advertising is used in many realms like medical fraternity. However, like in the business world, advertising in traditional medicine in southern Africa has met with a number of ethical quandaries and/or challenges. As revealed by the sampled data, the challenges met by traditional medicine have been largely a result of unethical techniques employed by traditional medical practitioners to advertise their products and services. It is in this light that I have argued that the 'diabolic' stance and derogatory connotations about the practice of traditional healing adopted in literature partly stems from an acoustic understanding of the practice and unethical advertising principles deployed by the practitioners themselves. This is compounded by the limitations of expert science to explicate the cosmology of the 'world beyond', and the conflation of witchcraft with traditional healing.[29] In this work, I have therefore demonstrated that the mounting incidences of unethical and morally unacceptable advertising strategies mire the whole practice of traditional healing with controversies. These incidences have proven beyond reasonable doubt that most traditional healers in southern African urban societies lack both business and medical ethics, hence the need for the national governments of countries concerned to work in cohorts with some independent organizations to empower and provide civic education to both the traditional healers and the public in general.

Most importantly, I have argued that ethics and its influence in business in general and medical fraternity in particular should not be underestimated. I underscored that any business, be it in medicine or elsewhere, can only gain credence and acceptance in society if it regards ethics. The merit of this work therefore lies in its quest to see to it that practitioners in spiritual healing and herbal medicine uphold ethical principles in ways that illuminate understanding of their practices.

Notes

1. Uk-skeptics, 'An overview of herbology: The use of herbs as medicine', 2004, Available online @ *http://www.timesonline.co.uk/article/02-1166505,00html,* (Accessed on 15/07/2011).

2. Olapade E.O. 'Preface', in E.O. Olapade (ed), *Traditional Medicine in Nigeria.* Lagos: Victoria Island, 1998.

3. Pretorius E. 'Traditional Healers'. *Unpublished manuscript.* University of the Orange Free State, 1992.

4. Ritchter M. 'Traditional Medicines and Traditional Healers in South Africa.' *Discussion Paper Prepared for the Treatment Action Campaign and AIDS Law Project.* 2003, 27 November:1-29.

5. Australian Journal of Medicinal Herbalism, "Blending science with tradition" Available online @ *(http://www.nhaa.org.au/index.php?),* (Accessed on 16/07/2011).

6. University of Maryland Medical center, "Herbal medicine", 2009, Available online @ *http://www.umm.edu/medref/,* (/Accessed on 12/05/2011).

7. University of Maryland Medical center, "Herbal medicine", 2009, Available online @ *http://www.umm.edu/medref/,* (/Accessed on 12/05/2011).

8. Grayson S. Spiritual healing: A simple guide for the healing of body, mind and spirit, Simon and Schuster Adult Publishing Group, 1997, Available online @ *http://www.stuartgrayson.com/index.html,* (Accessed 05/06/2011).

9. Church, D. (ed). *The heart of healing: Inspired ideas, wisdom and comfort from today's leading voices,* Elite Books, 2004, Available online @ dawson.church.comprar-livro.com.br/livros/1097200283/, (Accessed 16/07/2011).

10. Traditional Medicine Strategy, *World Health Organization,* Switzerland: Geneva, 2002-2005:7.

11. Pretorius, E. 'Traditional Healers'. *Unpublished manuscript.* University of the Orange Free State, 1992.

12. Ritchter, M. 'Traditional Medicines and Traditional Healers in South Africa.' *Discussion Paper Prepared for the Treatment Action Campaign and AIDS Law Project.* 2003, 27 November:1-29.

13. Offiong, D. A. Traditional Healers in the Nigerian Health Care Delivery System and the Debate over Integrating Traditional and Scientific Medicine. *Anthropological Quarterly* 72, 1999; (3): 118–130.

14. Adegoju, A. 'A Rhetorical Analysis of the Discourse of Advertising Herbal Medicine in South-western Nigeria'. *Linguistik Online* 2008, 33 (1/80):1-16. Available online @*http://www.linguistik-online.de/33_08/index.html,* (Accessed on 16/07/2011).

15. DeGeorge, R.T. Ethics *and Business,* Macmillan Publishing Company: London, 1982.

16. Mutungi, O.K. *The Legal Aspects of Witchcraft in East Africa with Particular Reference to Kenya.* Nairobi: East African Literature Bureau, 1977: xviii.

17. Pretorius, E. 'Traditional Healers'. *Unpublished manuscript*. University of the Orange Free State, 1992.

18. Ritchter, M. 'Traditional Medicines and Traditional Healers in South Africa.' *Discussion Paper Prepared for the Treatment Action Campaign and AIDS Law Project*. 2003, 27 November: 1-29.

19. Mawere, M. The Business of Business is Business?: The Myth of Amoral Business and Business Practices in Zimbabwe, *Journal of Social Development in Africa*, 2010; 25 (1): 271.

20. Iroegbu, P. Harvesting Knowledge of Herbal Resources and Development of Practitioners, *Indilinga: African Journal of Indigenous Knowledge Systems*, 2006; 5 (1) 32–50.

21. Adegoju, A. 'A Rhetorical Analysis of the Discourse of Advertising Herbal Medicine in South-western Nigeria'. *Linguistik Online* 2008, 33 (1/80):1-16. Available online @*http://www.linguistik-online.de/33_08/index.html*, (Accessed on 16/07/2011).

22. Fieser J. Do business have moral obligations beyond what the law requires?, *Journal of Business Ethics*, 1996; 15 (4): 457-468.

23. Mawere, M. The Business of Business is Business?: The Myth of Amoral Business and Business Practices in Zimbabwe, *Journal of Social Development in Africa*, 2010; 25 (1): 269-284.

24. Fieser J. Do business have moral obligations beyond what the law requires?, *Journal of Business Ethics*, 1996; 15 (4): 457-468.

25. Grice, P. H. 'Logic and Conversation', in P. Cole and J. Morgan (eds), *Syntax and Semantics: Volume 3, Speech Acts*. New York: Academic Press, 1975, p.43-58.

26. Leech G. *Principles of pragmatics*, Longman: London, 1993.

27. Harris M. and Seldon A, *Advertising and the Public*. Britain: Institute of Economic Affairs, 1962.

28. Norris, J. *Advertising*, Reston Publishing Company, 1980, p.413.

29. Mawere, M. Possibilities for cultivating African indigenous knowledge systems (IKSs): Lessons from selected cases of witchcraft in Zimbabwe, *Journal of Gender and Peace Development*, 2011;1 (3): 091-100.

Chapter Seven

Beneficence and Life Saving in Biomedicine

Medical ethics is a system of moral principles that apply values and judgments to the practice of medicine and as a scholarly discipline, it encompasses its practical application in clinical settings as well as work on its history, philosophy, theology, anthropology and sociology[1]. As such there are a number of values in medical ethics such as autonomy, non-maleficence, confidentiality, dignity, honesty, justice and beneficence, among others. These values act as guidelines for professionals in the medical fraternity and are therefore used to judge different cases in medicine. For purposes of this chapter, I will only focus on the principle of beneficence in biomedicine.

The Nature of the Principle of Beneficence

The concept of beneficence though widely used in medicine is difficult to define with precision. As such, a number of interpretations have been conjured. However broadly used in English, the word beneficence is considered to mean "the doing of good, the active promotion of good, kindness and charity"[2] or any action that is done for the benefit of others.[3] Though traditionally, acts of beneficence are often done from obligation, the principle is suggestive of altruism, humanity, unconditional love and nonobligatory optional moral ideals. More commonly in medical ethics, beneficence is understood as a principle requiring that physicians provide, and to the best of their ability, positive benefits such as good health, prevent and remove harmful conditions from patients. This is to say that beneficence as a principle of medical ethics asserts an obligation (on the part of the physician) to help others (patients) further their important and legitimate interests and abstain from injuring them in any way, that is, psychologically, morally or physically.

From the foregoing, it can be noted that the central question for beneficence within the patient-physician relationship is: "What does it mean for the physician to seek the greater balance of good over harm in the care of patients?"[4] The beneficence model answers this question at least in terms of the perspective that medicine takes on the patient's best interests rather than the physician's. The model clearly explicates that the central theme for beneficence is the physician's obligation to benefit patients. This has its earliest expression or its primary historical sources in ancient Greece and the Hippocratic Oath which characterizes physicians as a group of committed men (as women were excluded from medicine in the Greek society) set apart from and above others in the society. The central values of the classical Hippocratic ethics were nonmaleficence (doing no harm), beneficence and confidentiality. As such, the physician, according to the Hippocratic writings has always had the obligation to "apply dietetic measures to the benefit of the sick according to his ability and judgment, and he ought to keep patients from harms and injustice."[5]

In the modern era, the Hippocratic Oath is traceable to the 18th century with John Gregory and after World War II, medical ethics started to advocate patient autonomy in the guise of informed consent. However, over the last 20 years, there has been growing dissatisfaction with the individual rights-cantered ethical framework.[6] Yet like its old version, the Oath stresses on the virtues that keep the physician's attention fixed on his obligations to patients and the latter's best interests, rather than the physician's personal interests. Thus the Hippocratic Oath, by itself, is a "mere" skeleton of the principle of beneficence in so far as it sheds light on concepts that define what it means to be a physician and to 'benefit the sick' while avoiding 'harm and injustice'-the moral responsibility of physicians to do away with the sufferings of the sick, and to lessen the violence of their diseases.

The Complexities of Beneficence in Biomedicine

As has been seen on the nature of the principle of beneficence explicated above, the obligation to confer benefits and actively prevent and remove harms from patients is important in biomedical ethics. However, equally important is the obligation to assess or "weigh and balance the possible goods against the possible harms of an action."[7] This makes it important to distinguish two principles under the general principle of beneficence-the principle of positive beneficence and the principle of utility.[8] The first principle is known as the principle of positive beneficence. This principle requires the provision of benefits including the prevention and removal of harm from others (i.e. patients). It also includes the promotion of welfare of others. The second version is the principle of utility. This principle, unlike the first, requires weighing and balancing benefits and harms in moral life. This is to say that utility as a principle of beneficence in biomedical ethics makes it imperative for physicians and other health workers to carefully analyse, evaluate and promote those

133

actions that bring more benefits to others (i.e. patients) or the general public.

The second version makes it clear that the principle of beneficence is a *prima facie* moral obligation. For the moral philosopher, Ross, a *prima facie* principle is that "principle always to be acted upon unless it conflicts on a particular occasion with an equal or stronger principle."[9] In other words, a *prima facie* principle/obligation is that which sometimes is overridden when it conflicts with an equal or a stronger obligation; it is always right and binding, all other things being equal. In the real life situation, we must balance the demands of these principles by determining which carries more weight in the particular case. This is to say that a moral person's "actual" duty is always determined by weighing and carefully balancing all competing *prima facie* duties in any given situation. This means that the principle of beneficence is not absolute as it is not always binding. Yet this is where the complexity of the principle of beneficence begins in biomedicine. If the principle of beneficence is not absolute in biomedicine, it means that beneficence in biomedicine is not only restricted in application to the patient-physician relationship. It also extends to third parties to that relationship in so far as third parties to the patient-physician relationship can be affected, positively or otherwise. This means that while the physician, according to the principle of beneficence, has the obligation to prevent and remove harm from his/her patients the former can also harm third parties if the physician acts exclusively to benefit the patients. To make this clearer, let us consider the following situation:

In a particular city, X lives a couple, W and H. The husband P is HIV positive, but for fear of revealing this

134

information to his wife who is negative and pregnant decides to conceal this information to her. Instead, H sought to arrange a family medical Doctor who helps him with medication to prolong his life.

In this case, the third part, W (to the patient, H – physician relationship) is harmed if the family medical Doctor act exclusively to the benefit of his patient by concealing this information to W. This situation puts the Doctor in a very difficult position especially considering the right of patience to confidentiality. However, the principle of beneficence should be given priority over the principle of respect for patient confidentiality; we need to move beyond individual rights to common good. This is echoed by Margit Sutrop[10] who argues that defence of autonomy and privacy has become an obstacle not only to the use of data in scientific research but also to the use of such information in the implementation of social goals. For him, it has been claimed that epidemiological research is being obstructed, as statistical data cannot be collected without the subject's explicit agreement. Thus coming back to the example given above, respecting third part(ies) will be more desirable. In fact since the principle of beneficence is *prima facie* the second version of the principle- the principle of utility- would require that the third part, W be informed so that she and the foetus are not harmed (not infected as well). By doing so, the Doctor will have removed balanced and removed harms from the third parties (W and the foetus) though H's right to confidentiality will have been violated. Thus in this case, the principle to save more lives (of W and the foetus) is stronger than the right to confidentiality of H.

The Implications of Beneficence in Biomedicine

From the exposition of the nature and complexities of beneficence in the previous sections, it is sufficient to infer that the principle has a number of implications. As previously highlighted, the first principle under the general principle of beneficence- positive beneficence-imply beneficence even to third parties. Put it in other words, since the moral life does not permit us simply to produce benefits without creating risks, positive beneficence would imply that even the third parties to the relationship between the physician and the patient should be benefited. This, however, often creates ethical quandaries-moral dilemmas difficult to solve. One neat case is the example I have given in the previous section, that of a family medical Doctor who happens to know that one of the partners of his clients, H is HIV positive. The Doctor falls in a dilemma of whether s/he should conceal or disclose the information to the third partner (H's wife).

Second, the principle of utility under the general principle of beneficence implies that the interests of the society as a whole should override the individual interests and rights.[11] This implication if granted, can be interpreted to mean that in the context of medical research, for example, the principle entails that dangerous research on human subjects could be undertaken, and even ought to be undertaken, when the prospects of substantial benefits to society/majority outweighs the danger of the research to the individual. In the light of this analysis, the unconstrained principle would allow, for instance, a bone marrow transplant, which has the possibility of risks of the donor becoming a cripple or even dying, to be undertaken from a societal member to benefit a democratic president of a Republic who is suffering from an

136

end-stage organ failure. This example makes it clear that an unconstrained principle of utility carries danger (especially to the minority, unpopular or disadvantaged) with it since it implies that dangerous and sometimes immoral researches on human subjects "ought" to be undertaken. This is echoed by Gallap Survey who argues that the general principle of beneficence especially that with a version of the principle of utility implies that premature or hastened death of individual donors of cadaver organs done in order to benefit patients is justified.[12] Thus for Survey, the principle of utility shows that the principle would justify hastening death of one patient in order to benefit say five others who would procure a heart, a kidney, a liver, an eye and bone marrow each. This situation that beneficence implies is very problematic. It shows that the principle is prone to abuse. As a matter of consequence, unconstrained principle of beneficence generates a sense of distrust and fear for abuse in donors of cadaver organs as they would always worry that physicians might declare them dead prematurely in order to benefit other patients.

Another implication of beneficence has been cited by Peter Singer. He applies the principle in situations such as poverty. For Singer, since requirements of positive action are grounded in principles of preventing or acting to avoid bad outcomes, it implies that "obligatory/over-demanding beneficence requires that we should give until we reach a level at which by giving more, we would cause as much suffering to ourselves as we would relieve through our gift."[13] Put it differently, positive beneficence implies that we are morally obligated to make large sacrifices and substantially reduce our standard of living in an effort to rescue destitute or poor people around the world. The rich for example would be obliged to reduce their wealth to approximately the level of the poorest person in the world. In medical quarters, the health persons will be obliged to sacrifice their health in order to ameliorate the sick's situations. Thus, though the principle of beneficence is a *prima facie* some of the implications that arise especially in the medical fraternity and other spheres as a result of its presence make it problematic.

Overall, it can be argued that the principle of beneficence is fundamentally important in the preservation of life, in maximizing patients' well-being, in cost avoidance and risk reduction. Nevertheless, the principle like other ethical principles is fine in theory, but putting it into practice is more difficult as every situation is different.[14] This means that beneficence, as with other ethical issues in medicine should be approached on a case-by-case basis. Margit Sutrop hammering the same point argues that "although autonomy and beneficence seem at times to be in conflict, there is no reason to see one or the other as dominant."[15] This is because "both autonomy and beneficence as with other ethical principles are needed, but their specific interdependence depends on the particular situation and on social and political context."[16]

On Behalf of a Pragmatic and Rationalized Medical Ethic

Truth especially moral truth is certainly one of the hardest things to come by. It is hard enough to resolve rationally the moral and tradition based questions addressed in the preceding discussion. One would even think it's a waste of time to pursue such questions. To this kind of thinking, I disagree. I feel obliged to say that moral questions are not everyone's taste. It remains a truism that moral

138

curiosity and quest for understanding the good and the bad, the right and the wrong are a worthy and even sometimes a noble human characteristic. This is what David Hume meant when he correctly observed: "It is almost impossible for the mind of man to rest, like those of beasts, in that narrow circle of objects, which are the subject of daily conservation and action."[16] When we venture of such a narrow circle, we unavoidably bump into questions of moral/ethical nature; human beings can hardly eschew making some judgments about themselves, other human beings and the world. This exercise of making judgment is the beginning of moral reasoning.

Though acknowledging that euthanasia, physician strike, traditional medicine advertising and beneficence in biomedicine are contested terrains, this work has tried to make a judgment of these issues based on critical questioning and a "culture" of mutual negotiations. The work has exposed the different dimensions that these issues have assumed as they were constructed and evolved over the years in Africa and beyond. It is my conviction that the preceding discussion might not take us far toward a deep and comprehensive understanding of African medical ethics. However, I remain hopeful that enough has been said, at least, to help understand their underpinnings and judge how they can be reconstructed and carried on to posterity. More importantly is my fervent hope that enough has been said to encourage readers to take stock of their favoured views of euthanasia, strike, advertising and beneficence to seriously consider the possibility that the representation I made in this book may, in some respects, be in need of revision.

It goes without saying that mistakes are common. No doubt, my position in this book may contain mistakes and my own representation of the African world and the world in general is in a distressing number of ways incomplete and of course in many ways in transition and possible process of protection. I invite the reader to bring this to light. However, some of my moral beliefs paraded in this book seem to me both well-founded and unlikely to require revision. In view of African traditional culture, the work has emphasized that the "African view" and other such views on euthanasia, strike, advertising and beneficence advanced in this work are premised on mutual dependence, socialization into the values of a community (African communalism) and the biblical injunction "Do not kill."[17] In this respect, the book shares a classical tradition which stresses that euthanasia, physician strike, advertising and beneficence are public matters and not private choices insofar as they involve our conception of how we ought to live together in an ideal society. Public policy should therefore reflect on how citizens ought to behave and act.

It is also acknowledged that all that needs to be said on medical ethics and on Africa and beyond cannot be said in such a small text as this, but I believe the book has done enough "justice" to ignite more discussions and opened more windows through which burning issues in biomedicine can be viewed; to call for the reversal of African traditional views and Eurocentric paradigms of the selected issues where only pro- and con- arguments have remained the talk of the debate even in the present day. It is my fervent hope that such a bold step will revive the medical fraternity on issues to do with decision making on different cases/issues of biomedicine. It would set a good and illuminating example to the world and re-direct the debates on biomedicine to a common "fertile" ground that benefits all.

Notes

1. Wikipedia, 2010. 'Medical ethics,' Available online@ *http://en.wikipedia.org/wiki/medical_ethics#psearch. (*Accessed on 10 September 2011).

2. Beauchamp, T.L. Ed. Medical ethics: The moral responsibilities of physicians, Prentice-Hall: New Jersey, 1984, p.27.

3. Steven, P. 2008. 'Autonomy vs. Beneficence', Available online @ http://medschool.ucsf.edu/

4. Beauchamp, T.L. and Childress, J.F. Principles of biomedical ethics, 4rd ed. New York: Oxford University Press, 1994.p.28.

5. Jones, W.H.S. trans. Hippocrates 'Selections from the Hippocratic Corpus' In Veatch, R. M. ed. *Cross cultural perspectives in medical ethics*, J and Burllett Publishers: Boston, 1989, p.29.

6. Sutrop, M. 'Models of autonomy and beneficence', *Journal of Internal Medicine*, 2011; 269, p.375.

7. Beauchamp, T.L. ed. *Medical ethics: The moral responsibilities of physicians,* Prentice-Hall: New Jersey, 1989, p.195.

8. Beauchamp, T.L. ed. *Medical ethics: The moral responsibilities of physicians,* Prentice-Hall: New Jersey, 1989.

9. Ross, W.D. cited In Beauchamp, T.L. Ed. *Medical ethics: The moral responsibilities of physicians,* Prentice-Hall: New Jersey, 1989, p.14.

10. Sutrop, M. 'Models of autonomy and beneficence', *Journal of Internal Medicine*, 2011; 269, p.375–382.

11. Beauchamp, T.L. ed. *Medical ethics: The moral responsibilities of physicians,* Prentice-Hall: New Jersey, 1989.

12. Survey, G. "The US public's attitude toward organ transplant/organ donation", Journal of Contemporary Health Law and Policy, Princeton: New Jersey, p.1985.

13. Singer, P. Practical ethics, Cambridge University Press, 1979, p. 68.

14. Runzheimer, J. and Larsen, L.J. 2011. 'Reviewing Ethics and Common Controversies in Medicine,' Available online @http://www.dummies.com/search.html?

15. Sutrop, M. 2011. 'Models of autonomy and beneficence', *Journal of Internal Medicine*, 2011; 269, p.378.

16. Sutrop, M. 2011. 'Models of autonomy and beneficence', *Journal of Internal Medicine*, 2011; 269, p.378.

17. David Hume in *Treatise of Human Nature*, Oxford University Press, Oxford, England, 1960, p.271.

18. Exodus 20 v.13, *The Holly Bible, New International Version*, International Bible Society, Colorado, USA, 1984.